A
GUIDEBOOK
TO
NUTRITION

A Comprehensive guide to essential Vitamins, Minerals & Omega oils

INARA LEIGH

CONTENTS

INTRODUCTION

The human body is an incredibly complex piece of biological machinery capable of growth, development, adaptation, and countless other things.

Your body might seem inert, but thousands of biological processes occur daily, allowing you to feel, think, function, move, and live a healthy life. Even something as simple as raising your hand to your face requires complicated communication and signalling between your brain and body.

For these processes to occur, your body needs a wide range of nutrients, including protein, carbohydrates, dietary fats, vitamins, and minerals.

A SIMILARITY YOU MAY NEVER HAVE THOUGHT ABOUT.

Have you ever been to a gas station? If so, you've probably noticed that car fuel comes in several broad categories, each with a unique price per gallon.

The more expensive fuel is also higher quality, allowing the car to function optimally and last more miles. In contrast, lower-quality fuel is cheaper and thus more alluring.

The problem is that putting low-quality fuel in your car increases the risk of engine damage, poor performance, higher fuel consumption, and more. You can save some money on cheaper fill-ups, but it will eventually catch up with you.

Your body is similar in many ways. It needs high-quality fuel to run optimally and last serious mileage. Each nutrient carries out unique functions and contributes to your well-being, energy levels, cognitive function, and more.

You can get away with poor nutrition for a while, but a lousy diet opens the door to various health issues in the future.

THREE SOLID REASONS WHY NUTRITION IS CRUCIAL

1. It Makes You Feel Better

One of the biggest reasons for improving your nutrition is to feel better. Nourishing your body with the right foods promotes well-being in two major ways:

First, eating well is fulfilling and makes you feel great about yourself. In contrast, stuffing your body with junk food often feels good in the moment, but you end up feeling guilty afterward.

Second, nutritious foods provide the many nutrients your body needs to operate at peak efficiency. As a result, energy levels increase, cognition improves, and you're more motivated.

2. It Contributes to Optimal Growth and Development

It's no secret that nutrition fuels growth, but few people stop to consider the importance of a healthy diet.

Getting enough of all the essential nutrients is necessary for optimal growth and development in children and teenagers. Malnutrition is a significant issue that can contribute to impaired physical, mental, and intellectual development.

3. It Keeps You Healthy

Perhaps the biggest advantage of good nutrition is its impact on your health, well-being, and longevity. An ever-growing body of research suggests that our nutritional choices play a huge role in health outcomes and disease risk.

The Western diet, an eating approach based on processed food, is linked to:

- Obesity
- Cardiovascular disease
- Higher cancer rates
- Cognitive impairment
- Emotional disorders

In contrast, a healthy diet based on whole foods promotes a healthy weight, reduces the risk of various conditions, including heart disease and cancer, and contributes to a healthy state of mind.

People who primarily eat whole foods live longer, maintain a healthy weight, and are less likely to struggle with emotional eating and binge eating disorder.

VITAMIN A

Vitamin A is certainly not as popular as other nutrients like vitamins C and D, but the nutrient plays a vital role in our health.

In this chapter we'll go over vitamin A, share some surprising facts about the nutrient, review its many benefits, and more.

Read on to find out everything you need to know.

WHAT IS VITAMIN A?

Vitamin A refers to a group of identical nutrients your body needs to carry out many of its processes [1]. Retinol is the most popular, but we also have retinal and retinyl esters.

The A vitamins are fat-soluble and dissolve in organic solvents—substances with the capacity to dissolve various compounds [2]. Fat-soluble vitamins are absorbed alongside dietary fats and stored in the liver and fatty tissue.

Vitamin A is crucial for many bodily functions, some of which we'll explore in the following points. The two primary forms of vitamin A in food are preformed and provitamin. Preformed vitamin A is the active form of the nutrients, whereas provitamin A refers to the inactive form your body must first convert before using.

FIVE IMPRESSIVE HEALTH BENEFITS OF VITAMIN A

1. Immune System Support

The immune system is not some abstract entity that protects us from viruses and bacteria. It is the body's defense mechanism that determines how well you can fight off disease and stay healthy in the long run. Doing our best to maintain strong immunity is crucial for longevity, well-being, and good health.

Vitamin A is one of the nutrients responsible for your immune system. Some of its functions relate to the integrity of the mucous barriers in the gut, lungs, and eyes. These barriers trap invaders, preventing them from entering your body and promoting inflammation [3].

The collective of nutrients also plays a role in white blood cell production [4]. White blood cells, also known as leukocytes, are crucial fighters that protect your body from bacteria, viruses, and other harmful invaders. A low white blood cell count is linked to impaired immune system function.

2. Lower Risk of Acne

Acne is a significant problem that plagues millions of teenagers and adults. Despite being around forever, researchers and dermatologists still haven't found the optimal way to treat it.

Acne is considered a cosmetic problem, but that doesn't mean it cannot significantly impact a person's mental health and self-esteem. The skin condition can even lead to depression in some people [5].

One reason a person might struggle with acne is inadequate vitamin A intake. As discussed above, the nutrient is fat-soluble, which means the risk of deficiency is low. Still, it's possible for levels to drop, increasing the risk of skin problems.

A plausible mechanism for these effects is that low vitamin A levels lead to the overproduction of a protein called keratin within hair follicles [6]. As a result, dead skin is more challenging to eliminate and can block skin pores.

3. Promotes Healthy Bones

Bone health is crucial at any age, especially during childhood. Healthy bones promote optimal development and growth, allowing children to move freely and reach their full physical potential.

Three essential nutrients for bone health include protein, calcium, and vitamin D [7, 8]. But, according to research, having adequate vitamin A levels is also necessary for bone health [9]. The nutrient appears to be essential for the proper growth and development of our bones.

According to some data, low vitamin A levels are linked to lower bone mineral density and a higher risk of suffering from fractures [9]. Research also shows that people with higher vitamin A levels are at a lower risk of bone fractures [10].

It's important to note that researchers still don't fully understand the link between vitamin A levels and bone health. We need more research in the area, but preliminary data suggests that vitamin A and the nutrients mentioned above are vital for bone health.

4. Protects the Eyes and Vision

One of vitamin A's most notable health benefits is its ability to protect our eyes and vision. The nutrient's benefits related to sight and eye health are quite fascinating.

For one, vitamin A is a necessary component in converting light that reaches your eye into an electric signal that travels to your brain. One of the first symptoms of inadequate vitamin A levels is nyctalopia—night blindness; the inability to see in the dark [11].

The reason why vitamin A keeps nyctalopia is that it plays a vital role in producing rhodopsin (a pigment that is particularly sensitive to light and found in the retina of the eye). Adequate vitamin A levels lead to the optimal production of rhodopsin, reducing the risk of night blindness and allowing you to see better in the dark and in poorly lit rooms.

5. Potent Antioxidant Properties

Despite being seemingly inert, the human body is a powerhouse of metabolic activity. Each day, your body carries out thousands of metabolic processes related to energy expenditure, hormone synthesis, thinking, growth, and much more.

Most of the processes generate reactive oxygen species (ROS). These tiny and unstable molecules serve essential roles in the body, such as supporting immune system function and keeping us healthy [12].

Problems begin to occur when ROS levels become too high. At that point, these unstable molecules can damage healthy cells in the body and promote oxidative stress. Over time, that stress can put us at a higher risk of disease and early aging [13].

The body has an antioxidant system to prevent these adverse effects, but outside help is always welcome. Getting enough antioxidants through your diet leads to better health and lower disease risk.

As discussed above, one of the two primary vitamin A forms is provitamin A, which refers to a group of carotenoids (pigments). Despite not having the same activity as retinol, these compounds possess potent antioxidant properties and scavenge for reactive oxygen species [14].

VITAMIN A DOSAGE RECOMMENDATIONS AND SOURCES

The recommended daily allowance (RDA) of vitamin A is 900 mcg for men and 700 for women [15]. Children should consume slightly less [16]:

- 400 mcg daily for children aged 4 and 8
- 600 mcg daily for children aged 9 to 13

Teenagers can get close to the recommended doses for adults. The tolerable upper intake level (UL) is 3,000 mcg daily [15].

GREAT VITAMIN A SOURCES INCLUDE:

- Kale - 206 percent daily value per 100 grams
- Broccoli - 13 percent daily value per cooked cup
- Spinach - 64 percent daily value per cooked half-cup
- Carrots - 122 percent daily value per 100 grams cooked carrot
- Pumpkin - 60 percent daily value per cup of pureed pumpkin
- Sweet potato - 220 percent daily value per large, sweet potato
- Winter squash - 58 percent daily value per 100 grams
- Tomatoes - 11 percent daily value per medium-sized tomato
- Red bell pepper - 135 percent daily value per 100 grams
- Liver - 770 percent daily value per 100 grams
- Milk - 5 percent daily value per cup
- Eggs - 22 percent daily value per 100 grams (boiled)

As discussed, vitamin A comes in two primary forms: preformed (active) and provitamin (inactive). Some of the foods we listed provide an inactive form of vitamin A, which your body must first convert before use. Still, we've listed these in a simple format for you to understand how well each food can cover your daily needs.

THE DANGERS OF VITAMIN A DEFICIENCY

Vitamin A deficiencies are rare in developed countries but somewhat common in developing ones. A common reason for deficiencies in some parts of the world is the limited access to foods rich in preformed vitamin A and provitamin A.

According to data, vitamin A deficiency is the leading cause of vision loss in children worldwide [17]. Data also suggests that vitamin

A deficiency increases the risk of anemia and can have an adverse impact on fetal development during pregnancy [18]. A deficiency in the nutrient can also lead to more severe infections and a higher risk of fatal outcomes [19].

Vitamin A supplements can be helpful for certain groups of people, including pregnant and breastfeeding women and patients with cystic fibrosis. But, given that vitamin A is a fat-soluble nutrient, many people are concerned if supplementation leads to toxicities, so let's talk about that.

ARE THERE RISKS OF TOXICITIES?

The average person can meet their vitamin A needs by following a balanced diet based on whole foods. But, given that the average person eats fewer whole foods and more processed junk, many turn to supplements to cover their needs and prevent deficiencies.

As discussed earlier, vitamin A is a fat-soluble nutrient, which means we can store it inside fatty tissue and the liver for later use. Consuming too much of the nutrient can raise levels inside the body, bringing about toxicity.

The good news is that actual toxicities are relatively rare and are likely to occur in people who consume many vitamin A-rich foods while also supplementing with the nutrient.

CONCLUSION

Vitamin A is necessary for many bodily functions. The nutrient supports our health, prevents vision loss in children, and serves essential functions related to our immunity, skin health, and more.

Many foods provide some vitamin A, and the average person can cover their daily needs by following a healthy diet. A supplement can also be beneficial, but it's essential to avoid going overboard.

REFERENCES

1. www.ncbi.nlm.nih.gov/books/NBK482362/
2. www.ncbi.nlm.nih.gov/books/NBK218749/
3. www.pubmed.ncbi.nlm.nih.gov/6496388/
4. www.ncbi.nlm.nih.gov/pmc/articles/PMC6162863/
5. www.pubmed.ncbi.nlm.nih.gov/27799808/
6. www.longdom.org/open-access/role-of-diet-in-dermatological-conditions-2155-9600-1000400.pdf
7. www.pubmed.ncbi.nlm.nih.gov/21872800/
8. www.ncbi.nlm.nih.gov/pmc/articles/PMC4784773/
9. www.pubmed.ncbi.nlm.nih.gov/28891953/
10. www.pubmed.ncbi.nlm.nih.gov/24183637/
11. www.pubmed.ncbi.nlm.nih.gov/18806089/
12. www.ncbi.nlm.nih.gov/pmc/articles/PMC5551541/
13. www.ncbi.nlm.nih.gov/pmc/articles/PMC5927356/
14. www.ncbi.nlm.nih.gov/pmc/articles/PMC3942711/
15. www.ncbi.nlm.nih.gov/books/NBK222318/
16. www.lpi.oregonstate.edu/mic/life-stages/children
17. www.who.int/data/nutrition/nlis/info/vitamin-a-deficiency
18. www.ncbi.nlm.nih.gov/pmc/articles/PMC3843354/
19. www.pubmed.ncbi.nlm.nih.gov/24500929/

VITAMIN B3

Vitamin B3 is one of eight essential B vitamins with numerous vital roles in your body.

Today's chapter will go over precisely what the nutrient is, its benefits, what risks a deficiency can hide, and lots more.

Let's dive in.

WHAT IS VITAMIN B3?

Vitamin B3, also known as niacin, is one of the eight B vitamins your body needs for optimal health and well-being [1]. The two main forms of niacin are niacinamide (nicotinamide) and nicotinic acid. Both forms are similar in structure and effects on your body.

Like the other B vitamins, B3 is water-soluble, and any excess amounts get excreted through urination [1]. As such, we must get enough of the nutrient through food or supplements every day. Your body can also synthesize small amounts of niacin with the aid of an amino acid tryptophan found in milk, tuna, turkey, nuts, and other foods.

You might have heard that certain B vitamins are involved in hundreds of bodily processes [2]. One example of such a vitamin is B3. The nutrient plays a crucial role in synthesizing NAD (nicotinamide adenine dinucleotide) and NADP (nicotinamide adenine dinucleotide phosphate)—two coenzymes involved in roughly 400 biological processes [2].

Vitamin B3's main functions relate to extracting the energy from the foods we eat.

5 HEALTH BENEFITS OF OPTIMAL VITAMIN B3 LEVELS

1. Controls Blood Cholesterol Levels

One of niacin's functions in the body is to control blood lipid levels and promote cardiovascular health. The nutrient offers benefits on three fronts [3]:

- It lowers LDL (low-density lipoprotein) cholesterol
- It raises HDL (high-density lipoprotein) cholesterol
- It lowers blood triglyceride levels

Elevated LDL and blood triglycerides are linked to a higher risk of cardiovascular disease [4]. In contrast, HDL cholesterol is necessary for protecting the cardiovascular system by modulating inflammation and promoting cholesterol efflux (a process where excess cholesterol is transported to the liver for breakdown) [5].

Low HDL leads to a drop in cholesterol efflux, causing plaque to build up inside the blood vessels surrounding the heart and increasing the risk of a cardiovascular event [6].

It's important to note that such benefits appear when taking high niacin doses—typically over 1,500 mg daily [7].

2. Potential Benefits For Individuals With Type 1 Diabetes

Type 1 diabetes is a condition that affects people of all ages, including small children. The disease is characterized by chronically elevated blood sugar levels due to the pancreas' low or non-existent insulin production [8].

Researchers believe that type 1 diabetes is an autoimmune condition that results from the immune system attacking healthy cells by accident.

The attack permanently damages the pancreas, rendering the organ incapable of producing the hormone insulin.

There is currently no cure for diabetes, but treatment is available and mandatory for people with the condition.

According to some data, niacin can reduce the risk of type 1 diabetes in children predisposed to the condition [9].

3. Possible Benefits For Your Skin

Niacinamide (nicotinamide) is a form of vitamin B3 with several notable benefits for the skin. It is not the same as niacin, but your body can synthesize it naturally when vitamin B3 levels in the body rise.

Despite being different from vitamin B3, taking niacinamide can contribute to healthy levels of the nutrient and prevent a deficiency. The nutrient promotes the production of building blocks (keratin) that strengthen the skin and maintain its elastic properties [10]. Niacinamide is also crucial for keeping the skin moisturized and reducing damage from external factors, such as sun exposure [10].

Data suggests that topical application of niacinamide can reduce inflammation and help people treat eczema, acne, and more [10]. Further, a 2015 study suggested that taking 500 mg of niacinamide twice daily reduces the risk of nonmelanoma skin cancer in susceptible individuals [11].

4. Promotes Brain Function

The brain makes up roughly two percent of your body weight but accounts for approximately 20 percent of your total daily energy expenditure [12]. Due to its complex structure and continuous functions, the brain needs a steady energy supply to function optimally and remain healthy.

As discussed above, vitamin B3 is crucial for producing the coenzymes NAD and NADP, both of which are necessary for the brain. For instance, adequate NAD levels are linked to improved mitochondrial function and biogenesis [13].

Early findings also suggest that niacin can slow down the progression of Alzheimer's disease, though the data is mixed [14].

5. It Can Contribute to a Healthy Blood Pressure

According to statistics, heart disease is a leading cause of mortality worldwide, accounting for nearly 700,000 deaths in the US alone [15]. High blood pressure, also known as hypertension, is a significant risk factor for cardiovascular disease and early death [16].

Another way niacin can offer cardiovascular protection is by regulating blood pressure. One of the vitamin's functions is to release prostaglandins––a group of lipids with numerous essential roles, including controlling blood flow. These nutrients can help blood vessels widen, allowing blood to flow more freely, leading to a drop in blood pressure [17].

Hypertension is often called the silent killer because most people don't experience noticeable symptoms. Unfortunately, a lack of symptoms doesn't mean everything is okay.

Still, we need more human research to fully understand niacin's effects on blood pressure and the exact mechanisms.

THE OPTIMAL VITAMIN B3 DOSAGE AND THE BEST SOURCES

The Food and Nutrition Board (FNB) in the United States defines 1 NE as 1 mg of niacin or 60 mg of the amino acid tryptophan [2]. As discussed above, the body can use tryptophan to synthesize some amount of the active niacin.

According to the same resource, the recommended daily intake of vitamin B3 is as follows [2]:

- First six months of life - 2 mg
- 7 to 12 months - 4 mg NE
- 1 to 3 years - 6 mg NE

- 4 to 8 years - 8 mg NE
- 9 to 13 years - 12 mg NE
- 14+ years - 16 mg NE (boys); 14 mg NE (girls)
- Pregnant and lactating women should consume 18 mg NE or 17 mg NE, respectively

Eating a healthy and balanced diet is the best way to get enough vitamin B3. Topical solutions can be beneficial for skin-related issues, but it would be challenging to calculate what amount of the nutrient you're truly getting. Supplements are also an option, but it would be best to take them under a doctor's supervision to treat a deficiency.

With that in mind, here is a list of foods rich in vitamin B3 and their respective amounts per standard serving (usually three ounces):

- Beef - 26 to 39 percent daily value
- Pork - 39 to 45 percent daily value
- Liver - 91 to 100 percent daily value
- Poultry - 70 to 83 percent daily value
- Tuna - over 100 percent daily value (per can)
- Salmon - 53 to 61 percent daily value
- Peanut butter - 25 to 30 percent daily value (per two tablespoons)
- Green peas - 20 to 24 percent daily value (per cup)
- Brown rice - 18 to 21 percent daily value (per cooked cup)
- Potato - 25 to 30 percent daily value per large potato

IS THERE A RISK OF VITAMIN B3 DEFICIENCY?

A niacin deficiency is highly unlikely because the nutrient occurs naturally in many animal and plant foods [2]. Niacin is also readily absorbed from most foods except certain cereals because it can be bound to insoluble fibers that pass through the GI tract.

Even people following more restrictive diets like carnivore or plant-based will be able to get the bare minimum. The only cases of a deficiency in the nutrient seem to occur in developing countries due to malnutrition, typically as a result of an underlying health issue related to alcohol abuse or the liver [2].

A vitamin B3 deficiency can lead to:
- Skin rashes and discoloration
- Fatigue
- Headaches
- Loss of appetite
- Cognitive issues and memory loss
- Impaired gut motility leading to diarrhea or constipation
- Depression

The problem with the associated symptoms is that each is common with other deficiencies and issues. Sometimes, you might experience these symptoms even if everything is okay, and the only accurate way to diagnose a niacin deficiency is to have blood work done.

HOW LIKELY IS A VITAMIN B3 TOXICITY (AND WHAT ARE THE CONSEQUENCES)

There is no real danger of vitamin B3 toxicity when following a healthy diet. Even larger doses don't seem to lead to health issues.

The only people who should be careful with their niacin intake are those taking a supplement. Some products offer large doses of the nutrient per dose and combining supplementation with a diet rich in vitamin B3 can cause issues. Nicotinamide doses of 3,000 mg or more per day can bring about side effects, including nausea, vomiting, and signs of liver toxicity [2, 18].

FINAL WORDS

Niacin is one of the eight B vitamins your body needs to function optimally. The good news is that a deficiency is unlikely to occur unless there is an underlying medical condition. Plenty of foods include some amounts of the nutrient, and the body absorbs it readily.

It's always best to consult your doctor if you suspect you might not be getting enough of the nutrient and are considering supplementation for yourself or your children.

REFERENCES

1. www.ncbi.nlm.nih.gov/books/NBK526107/
2. www.ods.od.nih.gov/factsheets/Niacin-HealthProfessional/
3. www.pubmed.ncbi.nlm.nih.gov/12873710/
4. www.ncbi.nlm.nih.gov/pmc/articles/PMC6585375/
5. www.nature.com/articles/nrcardio.2010.222
6. www.ncbi.nlm.nih.gov/pmc/articles/PMC4148835/
7. www.ncbi.nlm.nih.gov/pmc/articles/PMC4829575/
8. www.cdc.gov/diabetes/basics/what-is-type-1-diabetes.html
9. www.pubmed.ncbi.nlm.nih.gov/23231526/
10. www.pubmed.ncbi.nlm.nih.gov/17147561/
11. www.pubmed.ncbi.nlm.nih.gov/26488693/
12. www.ncbi.nlm.nih.gov/pmc/articles/PMC124895/
13. www.ncbi.nlm.nih.gov/pmc/articles/PMC6787556/
14. www.sciencedirect.com/science/article/abs/pii/S0197458012006203?via%3Dihub
15. www.cdc.gov/nchs/fastats/leading-causes-of-death.htm
16. www.bhf.org.uk/informationsupport/conditions/cardiovascular-heart-disease
17. www.pubmed.ncbi.nlm.nih.gov/33404619/
18. www.nap.nationalacademies.org/catalog/6015/dietary-reference-intakes-for-thiamin-riboflavin-niacin-vitamin-b6-folate-vitamin-b12-pantothenic-acid-biotin-and-choline

VITAMIN B6

Vitamin B6 is a crucial nutrient related to energy metabolism, mental health, immunity, and more.

Today's chapter will teach you what vitamin B6 is, how it works, what benefits it offers, and everything else you need to know.

Let's dive in and explore.

WHAT IS VITAMIN B6?

Vitamin B6, also known as pyridoxine, is one of the eight B vitamins the human body needs for optimal health and well-being [1]. Like the other B vitamins, B6 is water-soluble, and excess amounts are excreted through urine. As such, we need to get enough of the nutrient through food and supplements daily to avoid a deficiency.

Pyridoxine's primary functions relate to our metabolism and central nervous system [2]. The nutrient facilitates energy extraction from foods and aids neurotransmitter production [3].

Despite being a single nutrient, vitamin B6 plays a role in over 100 bodily processes and enzymatic reactions. Its most notable functions relate to the breakdown of macronutrients (proteins, carbs, and fats) for energy. Pyridoxine is also vital during pregnancy as it promotes healthy development and can reduce nausea [1, 4].

THE IMPORTANCE OF VITAMIN B6 FOR HUMAN HEALTH

1. Plays an Important Role in Our Immune System

The immune system is a complex network of cells, vessels, proteins, and organs that works all the time to protect your body from external invaders. Optimal immune system function is necessary for more than just dealing with the common cold. It is also essential for fighting viruses and protecting you from diseases, including cancer [5].

Numerous things can strengthen your immunity. Among these, we have optimal sleep, regular physical activity, and stress management [6, 7]. Good nutrition is also crucial for your immunity because the body's defense system needs large amounts of certain nutrients to function at its best [8].

Vitamin B6 is one of several nutrients we need to get through food and supplements to keep our immune system strong. According to research, a vitamin B6 deficiency can weaken the immune system, making the organism more susceptible to illness [9, 10]. Data also suggests that vitamin B6 supplementation can improve the immune response in critically ill patients [11].

2. Protective Effects Against Mental Conditions Like Depression

The brain needs a wide range of neurotransmitters (chemical messengers) to function optimally, allowing us to lead rich and fulfilling lives.

Vitamin B6 plays a vital role in mental health because it is necessary for the production of certain neurotransmitters, including dopamine, gamma-aminobutyric acid (GABA), and serotonin [12]. For instance, research suggests that low serotonin could be a significant contributor to unhappiness and major depression [13].

Some research also notes that vitamin B6 could play an important role in reducing blood levels of homocysteine—an amino acid linked to depression and other mental conditions [14].

Further, data finds a link between lower vitamin B6 levels and a higher risk of depression in elderly individuals [15].

Interestingly, some research doesn't find a benefit to vitamin B6 supplementation. In one observational study on people without depression, supplementing with B6, B9, and B12 didn't lead to a reduced risk of depressive symptoms [16].

3. Necessary for Reducing the Risk Of Anemia

Anemia is characterized by a lower-than-normal red blood cell count, resulting in reduced blood oxygen levels [17]. Common symptoms associated with anemia include pale skin, severe muscle weakness, fatigue, shortness of breath, brain fog, and sleepiness.

Sadly, the condition can also affect children. An estimated 20 percent of children in the US will be diagnosed with anemia at some point [18].

Adequate vitamin B6 levels can be beneficial in preventing anemia. The nutrient plays a vital role in producing hemoglobin—a protein that carries oxygen molecules throughout the body [19]. Low hemoglobin levels mean your body cannot carry oxygen to all cells, which leads to the symptoms mentioned above: weakness, fatigue, shortness of breath, etc.

The hypothesis makes sense because data links inadequate vitamin B6 levels with anemia, especially in pregnant women [20]. The only roadblock is that vitamin B6 deficiencies are relatively rare, and studying the supplement as a form of treatment is challenging.

One study found that giving pregnant women 75 mg of vitamin B6 daily reduced anemia symptoms [20].

4. It May Promote Eye Health and Good Vision

One hypothesis suggests that adequate vitamin B6 levels can promote eye health and good vision by controlling homocysteine. As mentioned above, the nutrient is necessary for controlling the amino acid because it can break down excess amounts to create other compounds your body needs.

Aside from increasing the risk of dementia, stroke, and mental conditions, chronically elevated homocysteine levels can increase the risk of age-related macular degeneration (AMD) [21].

The hypothesis suggests that since vitamin B6 controls levels of the amino acid, ingesting enough can reduce the risk of macular degeneration and promote good vision. Luckily, an observational study that tracked over 5,000 women for seven years suggested the idea to be true. According to the data, women that took a daily supplement consisting of vitamins B6, B9, and B12 were at a much lower risk of AMD [22].

Of course, it is difficult to say if vitamin B6 made the difference or if these findings were thanks to the combination of the three vitamins. But, given the nutrient's mechanisms, the idea makes sense.

5. Beneficial for Cardiovascular Health

Cardiovascular disease is one of the leading causes of death today [23]. It accounts for nearly 700,000 deaths annually and contributes to poor quality of life for millions worldwide.

While numerous factors, including your nutrition, sleep, and exercise habits, play a role in heart health, some data suggests that vitamin B6 can also help. Observational research suggests that people with low levels of the nutrient are at a much higher risk of coronary artery disease [24].

One potential mechanism behind these effects could be that vitamin B6 breaks down excess homocysteine. Chronically elevated levels of the amino acid are linked to cardiovascular disease and stroke [25, 26].

One study from 2000 had some interesting findings. In it, researchers gathered 158 siblings of people with a premature atherothrombotic disease and split them into two groups [27]. One group received 5 mg of vitamin B9 and 250 mg of vitamin B6 daily for two years; the other group received a placebo. Following the trial, the subjects that received the vitamin treatment had much lower homocysteine levels and much better cardiovascular markers.

HOW MUCH VITAMIN B6 DO YOU NEED, AND WHAT ARE SOME GOOD SOURCES?

Here are the recommended daily vitamin B6 intakes based on age [28]:

- First six months - 0.1 mg
- 7 to 12 months - 0.3 mg
- 1 to 3 years - 0.5 mg
- 4 to 8 years - 0.6 mg
- 9 to 13 years - 1 mg
- 14 to 18 years - 1.3 mg for boys, 1.2 mg for girls
- 19 to 50 years - 1.3 mg
- 51+ years - 1.7 mg for men, 1.5 mg for women
- Pregnant and lactating women should ingest 1.9 and 2 mg, respectively

There are many natural food sources of vitamin B6. Supplements and fortified foods are also available. Here are some of the best nutritional options with their respective amounts:

- Pork chops - 54 percent daily value per 6 ounces
- Chicken breast - 92 percent daily value per 6 ounces
- Salmon - 94 percent daily value per 6 ounces
- Beef - 48 percent daily value per 6 ounces
- Pistachio nuts - 28 percent daily value per ounce
- Bananas - 30 percent daily value per large banana
- Avocado - 30 percent daily value per avocado
- Potato - 32 percent daily value per medium-sized potato
- Sweet potato - 35 percent daily value per cup
- Fortified tofu - 66 percent daily value per cup

IS THERE A RISK OF VITAMIN B6 DEFICIENCY?

A vitamin B6 deficiency can harm your health, but the risk of developing one is low. Most people can get enough vitamin B6 by following a balanced diet. Similar to other B vitamins, even more restrictive dietary approaches (such as plant-based eating) can allow you to get enough of the nutrient to optimize your health.

Due to the small number of vitamin B6 deficiency cases, research on it is limited. Some data suggests that lower vitamin B6 levels can increase the risk of depression in older adults [29, 30]. A deficiency in the nutrient is also associated with other conditions in the elderly, including Alzheimer's, cardiovascular disease, and cancer [31].

HOW LIKELY IS VITAMIN B6 TOXICITY, AND WHAT ARE THE ASSOCIATED RISKS?

Like with other B vitamins, there is no risk of toxicity from food intake alone. Even a diet rich in vitamin B6 isn't likely to lead to dangerously high levels, given that the nutrient is water-soluble and your body excretes excess amounts through urine.

Supplementation with vitamin B6 has been shown to cause neuropathy (damage to the peripheral nervous system) [32]. Fortunately, these effects occur at doses of 1,000 mg per day or over 800 times the amount you can get from food.

CONCLUSION

Pyridoxine is a water-soluble nutrient and part of the B complex. The nutrient occurs naturally in many foods, and the risk of a deficiency is low. Toxicity is also rare unless a person takes large doses in supplement form.

Getting enough vitamin B6 is crucial for strong immunity, mental health, cardiovascular protection, and more.

REFERENCES

1. www.ncbi.nlm.nih.gov/books/NBK557436/
2. www.ncbi.nlm.nih.gov/pmc/articles/PMC6257116/
3. www.ncbi.nlm.nih.gov/pmc/articles/PMC6071262/
4. www.pubmed.ncbi.nlm.nih.gov/16625530/
5. www.ncbi.nlm.nih.gov/pmc/articles/PMC5091071/
6. www.ncbi.nlm.nih.gov/pmc/articles/PMC3256323/
7. www.ncbi.nlm.nih.gov/pmc/articles/PMC6523821/
8. www.ncbi.nlm.nih.gov/pmc/articles/PMC6723551/
9. www.ncbi.nlm.nih.gov/pmc/articles/PMC5358464/
10. www.pubmed.ncbi.nlm.nih.gov/8302491/
11. www.pubmed.ncbi.nlm.nih.gov/16670691/
12. www.ncbi.nlm.nih.gov/pmc/articles/PMC4288272/
13. www.ncbi.nlm.nih.gov/pmc/articles/PMC5302148/
14. www.pubmed.ncbi.nlm.nih.gov/17541043/
15. www.pubmed.ncbi.nlm.nih.gov/18838531/
16. www.pubmed.ncbi.nlm.nih.gov/18557664/
17. www.nhlbi.nih.gov/health/anemia
18. www.cedars-sinai.org/health-library/diseases-and-conditions---pediatrics/a/anemia-in-children.html
19. www.ncbi.nlm.nih.gov/books/NBK470579/
20. www.pubmed.ncbi.nlm.nih.gov/19920848/
21. www.pubmed.ncbi.nlm.nih.gov/14700648/
22. www.ncbi.nlm.nih.gov/pmc/articles/PMC2648137/
23. www.cdc.gov/nchs/fastats/leading-causes-of-death.htm
24. www.pubmed.ncbi.nlm.nih.gov/17045461/
25. www.pubmed.ncbi.nlm.nih.gov/9509248/
26. www.ncbi.nlm.nih.gov/pmc/articles/PMC5120102/
27. www.pubmed.ncbi.nlm.nih.gov/10683000/
28. www.ods.od.nih.gov/factsheets/VitaminB6-HealthProfessional/
29. www.pubmed.ncbi.nlm.nih.gov/18838531/

30. www.pubmed.ncbi.nlm.nih.gov/15479988/
31. www.pubmed.ncbi.nlm.nih.gov/17260529/
32. https://pubmed.ncbi.nlm.nih.gov/16320662/

VITAMIN B9

Vitamin B9 is an essential nutrient most people link to a healthy pregnancy. While the nutrient plays a crucial role in fetal development, its functions run far deeper than most people imagine.

Today's chapter will teach you everything you need to know about vitamin B9, its benefits, what foods you should eat, and much more.

Let's discuss.

WHAT IS VITAMIN B9?

Vitamin B9, also known as folate, is one of eight naturally occurring B vitamins, collectively known as the B complex [1]. Like all other B vitamins, folate is water-soluble, and your body does not store excess amounts for later use. As such, you must get enough of the nutrient through food every day.

Folate is a term that refers to similar compounds with identical effects on the body [1]. Most forms of the nutrient get converted to 5-methyltetrahydrofolate (5-MTHF) in your digestive system before entering the bloodstream [2].

The term folate comes from the Latin folium, which translates to leaf.

Folic acid (pteroylmonoglutamic acid) is the synthetic form of the vitamin, and people often use the two terms interchangeably. The compound is used in dietary supplements and is added to various foods [3].

Unlike folate, folic acid doesn't get fully converted to 5-MTHF in the digestive system [4]. Some of it needs to travel to the liver to be converted, and the process isn't as efficient for everyone [5]. As such, supplementation might not be as effective as getting the nutrient through food.

One study suggests that taking folic acid as part of a B complex supplement can make the conversion more efficient [6]. Doing so can reduce the risk of unmetabolized folic acid remaining in the bloodstream.

THE BENEFITS AND FUNCTIONS OF VITAMIN B9

1. A Vital Contributor to Healthy Pregnancy

Congenital disabilities were a mystery until a few decades ago. Researchers and medical professionals couldn't understand why some babies were born completely healthy, and others suffered from defects related to the brain or spine.

Researchers later discovered the crucial link between folate and congenital disabilities. Mothers with low levels of specific vitamins were more likely to give birth to babies with spina bifida (spinal defects) [7]. Eventually, large human trials showed that women taking folic acid or consuming more folates were at a much lower risk of giving birth to babies with congenital disabilities [8, 9].

In fact, folate is so crucial for a healthy pregnancy that women of childbearing age are advised to take a folic acid supplement [10]. Additionally, the FDA in the US requires that food manufacturers add folic acid to enriched pasta, rice, gains, and other products [10].

2. Contributes to a Healthy Brain

Homocysteine is an amino acid that results from various bodily processes. Elevated levels of the compound are linked to cognitive decline and a higher risk of Alzheimer's and dementia [11].

According to research, homocysteine can impact the brain by reducing blood flow to nerve cells [12].

Vitamins B6, B9, and B12 break down homocysteine to create other chemicals your body needs. Elevated homocysteine levels can indicate a deficiency in these three B vitamins [13, 14].

Some research also links low folate levels in the blood with a higher risk of dementia and Alzheimer's disease [15, 16].

3. It Might Reduce the Risk of Stroke

A stroke is a debilitating and life-threatening medical condition that restricts blood flow to a specific brain region. The result is damage to the brain that can lead to impediments or death.

According to data, over 12 million people suffer from a stroke each year, and more than half die as a result [17].

Just as homocysteine increases the risk of cognitive decline and neurological disorders, it can also lead to a stroke [18]. The good news is that vitamins B6, B9, and B12 break down the amino acid, thus reducing the risk of a life-threatening medical emergency [13, 14].

A review of 30 studies with over 82,000 participants found that folic acid supplementation reduced the stroke risk by 10 percent [19].

4. It Plays a Role in Red Blood Cell Production

Red blood cells have the crucial role of carrying oxygen molecules from the lungs to every part of your body. Upon their return, these cells carry carbon dioxide to the lungs for us to exhale [20].

Unfortunately, red blood cell production can decrease for various reasons, resulting in red blood cell anemia. The condition typically leads to fatigue, brain fog, pale skin, sleepiness, and more.

Aside from affecting adults, anemia is common in children, with an estimated 20 percent of children in the US being diagnosed at some point [21].

According to research, getting enough folate in your diet or taking a folic acid supplement can prevent that. The nutrient is crucial for producing fully functional red blood cells and preventing megaloblastic anemia [22, 23].

5. Possible Cancer-Preventing Properties

Cancer is one of the leading causes of death and disability worldwide. According to data, cancer resulted in 10 million deaths in 2020 [24]. Unfortunately, these statistics aren't likely to improve soon, given the elusive nature of cancer.

There are countless varieties of the disease, each affecting people in different ways. To make matters worse, cancer can occur for various reasons, including genetic predisposition and environmental factors.

One potential risk factor for cancer is low folate status [25]. While research is yet to understand the relationship, ensuring an adequate folate intake can be beneficial in the long run.

HOW MUCH VITAMIN B9 DO YOU NEED (AND WHAT ARE SOME GOOD SOURCES)?

The recommended daily intake (RDI) of folate is listed as dietary folate equivalents (DFEs). The measurement unit was developed to provide a single recommendation that works for folate and folic acid [3].

Here are the RDIs for folate and folic acid based on age [3]:
- First six months - 65 mcg DFE
- 7 to 12 months - 80 mcg DFE
- 1 to 3 years - 150 mcg DFE
- 4 to 8 years - 200 mcg DFE
- 9 to 13 years - 300 mcg DFE
- 14+ years - 400 mcg DFE

Pregnant and breastfeeding women should consume up to 600 mcg DFE of folate and folic acid [3].

Here are some of the best folate sources and how much each provides based on the RDI for adults:

- Lentils - 90 percent of RDI per cup (cooked)
- Kale - 65 percent of RDI per cup (raw)
- Beef liver - 54 percent of RDI per 3-ounce serving (cooked)
- Avocado - 42 percent per medium-sized avocado (raw)
- Beets - 37 percent of RDI per cup
- Asparagus - 34 percent of RDI per half cup (cooked)
- Kidney beans - 33 percent of RDI per cup (cooked)
- Brussel sprouts - 24 percent of RDI per cup (raw)
- Spinach - 15 percent of RDI per cup (uncooked)
- Oranges - 14 percent of RDI per large orange
- Eggs - 6 percent of RDI per large egg

IS THERE A RISK OF A VITAMIN B9 DEFICIENCY, AND WHAT ARE THE ASSOCIATED SYMPTOMS?

Folate deficiency is uncommon and typically coexists with other deficiencies due to an underlying health issue, alcoholism, or something else [3]. As you saw in the previous point, plenty of foods contain at least some folate, so the risk of not getting enough of the nutrient is low.

The primary symptom of a folate deficiency is megaloblastic anemia [22]. It is characterized by the production of large and dysfunctional red blood cells incapable of carrying oxygen throughout the body [23]. The result is a perpetual state of fatigue, sleepiness, and muscle weakness.

Women with folate deficiency are at a higher risk of giving birth to babies with congenital disabilities. A low folate status can also increase the risk of premature birth and low birth weight [3].

The best way to prevent a deficiency is to follow a balanced diet of animal and plant foods. A folic acid supplement is typically recommended to pregnant women or those seeking to conceive.

HOW LIKELY IS A VITAMIN B9 TOXICITY?

Vitamin B9 toxicity is extremely unlikely in people following a regular diet and not taking a supplement. Even people taking a folic acid supplement (e.g., pregnant women) are unlikely to see dangerous elevations of the nutrient.

As discussed earlier, folate is water-soluble, and excess amounts get excreted through urine.

Unfortunately, that's not all. Some research indicates that unmetabolized folic acid can contribute to higher disease risk (including cancer) [24]. Unmetabolized means your body hasn't broken the substance down, and it lingers in your bloodstream.

The good news is that no research finds a direct link, and the hypothesis is based on observations [25].

CONCLUSION

Folate is a naturally occurring nutrient and one of the eight B vitamins that play a crucial role in metabolic health, DNA synthesis, fetal development, and more. Folic acid is the synthetic form of the nutrient and is available as a supplement or as part of fortified foods.

The nutrient plays a crucial role during pregnancy, promotes brain health, and can reduce the risk of stroke and certain cancers.

Luckily, many foods are rich in folate, and the risk of deficiency is extremely low.

REFERENCES

1. www.ncbi.nlm.nih.gov/pmc/articles/PMC3648733/
2. www.ncbi.nlm.nih.gov/pmc/articles/PMC4867132/
3. www.ods.od.nih.gov/factsheets/Folate-HealthProfessional/
4. www.pubmed.ncbi.nlm.nih.gov/17617936/
5. www.pubmed.ncbi.nlm.nih.gov/16441927/
6. www.pubmed.ncbi.nlm.nih.gov/25943647/
7. www.pubmed.ncbi.nlm.nih.gov/1015847/
8. www.thelancet.com/journals/lancet/article/PII0140-6736(91)90133-A/fulltext
9. www.pubmed.ncbi.nlm.nih.gov/1307234/
10. www.hsph.harvard.edu/nutritionsource/folic-acid/
11. www.pubmed.ncbi.nlm.nih.gov/11455131/
12. www.pubmed.ncbi.nlm.nih.gov/18725259/
13. www.ncbi.nlm.nih.gov/pmc/articles/PMC28491/
14. www.ncbi.nlm.nih.gov/pmc/articles/PMC4425139/
15. www.ncbi.nlm.nih.gov/pmc/articles/PMC1123448/
16. www.ncbi.nlm.nih.gov/pmc/articles/PMC8079632/
17. www.world-stroke.org/world-stroke-day-campaign/why-stroke-matters/learn-about-stroke
18. www.ncbi.nlm.nih.gov/pmc/articles/PMC5120102/
19. www.pubmed.ncbi.nlm.nih.gov/27528407/
20. www.ncbi.nlm.nih.gov/books/NBK539702/
21. www.cedars-sinai.org/health-library/diseases-and-conditions---pediatrics/a/anemia-in-children.html
22. www.pubmed.ncbi.nlm.nih.gov/15189115/
23. www.ncbi.nlm.nih.gov/books/NBK537254/
24. www.who.int/news-room/fact-sheets/detail/cancer
25. www.ncbi.nlm.nih.gov/pmc/articles/PMC2790187/

VITAMIN B12

Vitamin B12 is among the most popular nutrients, and research links it to numerous health benefits.

Today's chapter will teach you everything you need to know about the nutrient. We'll review some of its most prominent benefits, the deficiency risk, the necessity of supplementation, and good food sources.

Let's dive in.

WHAT IS VITAMIN B12?

Vitamin B12, also known as cobalamin, is one of eight B vitamins, collectively known as the B complex [1]. Like the other seven B vitamins, cobalamin is water-soluble, and excess amounts get excreted through urine. As such, you must consume enough of the nutrient through food each day to avoid a deficiency.

Your liver can store small amounts of B12 for up to four or five years, but you must still get enough of the nutrient regularly to stay healthy and feel great.

The vitamin plays several crucial roles in your body, including keeping your nervous system healthy and promoting red blood cell production [1]. Cobalamin is also necessary for DNA synthesis, and severe deficiencies are linked to DNA damage.

B12 is the largest and most complex vitamin and occurs naturally in animal products, such as meat and eggs.

THE FUNCTIONS AND BENEFITS OF VITAMIN B12

1. It Contributes to a Healthy Pregnancy

Vitamin B9 (folate) is the first nutrient that comes to mind when discussing pregnancy, but B12 is also essential. The nutrient is necessary for the baby's healthy development [2].

Low vitamin B12 levels in pregnant women are linked to a higher risk of neural tube defects, miscarriages, and premature births [3]. For instance, one study suggested that serum vitamin B12 levels in pregnant women were closely connected to the likelihood of giving birth to a baby with congenital disabilities [4].

2. It Can Reduce the Risk of Mental Conditions

Early findings suggest that vitamin B12 could play a huge role in mood regulation, well-being, and reducing the risk of depression. Unfortunately, the mechanisms behind these effects aren't yet fully understood, and we need more data to determine the precise impact of B12 on the brain and nervous system.

For instance, one likely explanation is that a vitamin B12 deficiency can lead to lower serotonin levels. The neurotransmitter plays a vital role in our mood, and a drop can increase the risk of depression [5, 6]. Data also supports vitamin B12 supplementation for treating depressive symptoms [7].

One study suggested that taking vitamin B12 with anti-depressant medication improves treatment outcomes for major depressive disorder (MDD) [8].

3. It Reduces the Risk of Anemia

Anemia is characterized by a low red blood cell count [9]. Red blood cells play a crucial role in carrying oxygen molecules from the lungs to every part of the body [10]. These cells also transport carbon dioxide to the lungs for us to exhale.

A drop in red blood cell production can result from many things, including a nutrient deficiency [11]. The result is extreme fatigue, brain fog, loss of motivation to do anything, sleepiness, and similar.

Unfortunately, anemia can also affect children, and data shows that one in five children in the US will be diagnosed with the condition at some point [12].

The good news is that adequate vitamin B12 levels reduce the risk of anemia because they play an essential role in red blood cell production [13]. Iron and folate also play a crucial role in the process.

According to some sources, a vitamin B12 deficiency causes the body to produce larger red blood cells that cannot carry out their functions effectively [14]. The condition is called megaloblastic anemia.

4. It's Beneficial for Bone Health

Most people link calcium and potassium with optimal bone health. While the two minerals play an important role in bone mineral density, they are far from the only nutrients your body needs.

According to research, maintaining healthy vitamin B12 levels could be important for healthy bones. For instance, data finds a correlation between low B12 levels and lower bone mineral density in otherwise healthy people [15].

Other papers also find a correlation between lower vitamin B12 levels and a drop in bone mineral density [16, 17]. The connection appears to be particularly pronounced in women.

The biggest issue is that low bone mineral density increases the risk of fractures and the onset of osteoporosis—a debilitating condition often diagnosed after a fracture [18].

5. It Can Promote Brain Function and Health

Vitamin B12 appears to be beneficial for brain health in several ways. To understand one of the mechanisms, we must backtrack a bit and talk about homocysteine—an amino acid that can lead to serious health issues.

Homocysteine is the metabolic by-product of certain bodily processes. Under normal circumstances, vitamins B6, B9, and B12 break it down to produce other chemicals your body needs [19, 20]. But, when levels of these nutrients decrease, homocysteine metabolism slows down, and the amino acid is free to inflict damage.

One significant issue with homocysteine is that it reduces blood flow to the brain and nerve cells [21]. This is thought to be one mechanism by which the amino acid increases the risk of stroke. Additionally, the amino acid is linked to mental decline and a higher risk of dementia and Alzheimer's disease [22, 23].

Maintaining healthy vitamin B12 levels is necessary for keeping homocysteine levels low and preventing it from wreaking havoc on your health.

HOW MUCH VITAMIN B12 DO WE NEED, AND WHAT ARE SOME GOOD SOURCES?

Vitamin B12 needs vary by age, lifestyle, and health status. Here are the recommended daily intakes (RDI) by age [24]:

- 0 to 6 months - 0.4 mcg
- 7 to 12 months - 0.5 mcg
- 1 to 3 years - 0.9 mcg
- 4 to 8 years - 1.2 mcg
- 9 to 13 years - 1.8 mcg

- 14+ years - 2.4 mcg

Pregnant and breastfeeding women should increase their intake to 2.6 and 2.8 mcg per day, respectively [24].

Here are some of the best food sources of the nutrient and the respective quantities with regards to the RDI for adults:

- Lamb, beef, and veal liver meat - 3,000+ percent daily needs per 3.5 ounces
- Sardines - 500+ percent daily needs per cup (drained)
- Tuna - 400+ percent daily needs per 3.5 ounces
- Trout - 300+ percent daily needs per 3.5 ounces
- Beef - 245 percent daily needs per 3.5 ounces
- Salmon - 116 percent daily needs per 3.5 ounces
- Whole milk - 46 percent daily needs per cup
- Eggs - 23 percent daily needs per medium egg

Eating enough foods rich in vitamin B12 is vital because we don't seem the absorb the nutrient well from supplements [25].

IS THERE A RISK OF A VITAMIN B12 DEFICIENCY?

Healthy people are at low risk of a vitamin B12 deficiency simply because the nutrient is found in many everyday foods. People at risk of such a deficiency typically struggle with an underlying health issue that prevents them from absorbing nutrients adequately [24].

A significant problem that can develop due to a vitamin B12 deficiency is megaloblastic anemia [24]. The body produces abnormally large red blood cells that cannot carry out their functions effectively [14]. As a result, people with the condition experience extreme tiredness, fatigue, sleepiness, paleness, and similar symptoms.

As discussed earlier, low vitamin B12 can also increase the risk of neurological and mental conditions like dementia and depression [5, 6, 26].

Women with lower vitamin B12 levels are also at risk of premature birth and having a baby with congenital disabilities [2, 3, 4].

Older individuals and those suffering from gastrointestinal issues or pernicious anemia are at a higher risk of a vitamin B12 deficiency [24].

HOW LIKELY ARE WE TO EXPERIENCE VITAMIN B12 TOXICITY?

There isn't an established upper limit for vitamin B12 because the risk of toxicity is incredibly low. Vitamin B12 is a water-soluble nutrient, and excess amounts get excreted through urine.

Additionally, people following a varied diet are unlikely to consume that much of the nutrient on any given day. Organ meat and certain fish are rich in B12, but most people don't eat these foods daily.

Supplementing with extremely high doses can lead to some issues, including acne and other skin issues, and health complications in people with chronic conditions like type 2 diabetes [27, 28].

The best way to avoid potential issues is to follow a healthy and balanced diet. Supplementation is necessary for some people, but it's best to consult your doctor and take a supplement under their supervision.

FINAL WORDS

Vitamin B12 is one of the eight essential B vitamins, collectively known as the B complex. Like the other B vitamins, B12 is water-soluble, and excess amounts are excreted through urine.

The risk of vitamin B12 toxicity is low, but you should eat a balanced diet to avoid a deficiency. People following a vegan diet and those dealing with an underlying condition can consider supplementation after consulting their healthcare provider.

Adequate levels of the nutrient are necessary for a healthy pregnancy, mental health, strong bones and teeth, brain function, and reducing the risk of anemia.

REFERENCES

1. www.ncbi.nlm.nih.gov/books/NBK559132/
2. www.ncbi.nlm.nih.gov/pmc/articles/PMC8074968/
3. www.pubmed.ncbi.nlm.nih.gov/18709885/
4. www.ncbi.nlm.nih.gov/pmc/articles/PMC4161975/
5. www.ncbi.nlm.nih.gov/pmc/articles/PMC4728667/
6. www.ncbi.nlm.nih.gov/pmc/articles/PMC5302148/
7. www.ncbi.nlm.nih.gov/pmc/articles/PMC3856388/
8. www.pubmed.ncbi.nlm.nih.gov/14641930/
9. www.ncbi.nlm.nih.gov/books/NBK499994/
10. www.ncbi.nlm.nih.gov/books/NBK539702/
11. www.ncbi.nlm.nih.gov/pmc/articles/PMC6697587/
12. www.cedars-sinai.org/health-library/diseases-and-conditions---pediatrics/a/anemia-in-children.html
13. www.pubmed.ncbi.nlm.nih.gov/15189115/
14. www.ncbi.nlm.nih.gov/books/NBK537254/
15. www.pubmed.ncbi.nlm.nih.gov/15619681/
16. www.pubmed.ncbi.nlm.nih.gov/12612156/
17. www.pubmed.ncbi.nlm.nih.gov/19151987/
18. www.ncbi.nlm.nih.gov/books/NBK441901/
19. www.ncbi.nlm.nih.gov/pmc/articles/PMC4425139/
20. www.ncbi.nlm.nih.gov/pmc/articles/PMC28491/
21. www.pubmed.ncbi.nlm.nih.gov/18725259/
22. www.ncbi.nlm.nih.gov/pmc/articles/PMC8079632/
23. www.ncbi.nlm.nih.gov/pmc/articles/PMC1123448/
24. www.ods.od.nih.gov/factsheets/VitaminB12-HealthProfessional/
25. www.ashpublications.org/blood/article/112/6/2214/24841/How-I-treat-cobalamin-vitamin-B12-deficiency
26. www.ncbi.nlm.nih.gov/pmc/articles/PMC7077099/
27. www.pubmed.ncbi.nlm.nih.gov/25559140/
28. www.pubmed.ncbi.nlm.nih.gov/20424250/

VITAMIN C

We are all familiar with vitamin C. Most people know it as the nutrient found in oranges that also comes in dissolvable tablet form we can take when dealing with the common cold.

While the nutrient can undoubtedly be helpful when dealing with the cold or flu, its effects on the body are far more profound.

To that end, Let's go over vitamin C and outline five of the best benefits for people of all ages. We'll also discuss dosage guidelines, good sources of the nutrient, and hidden dangers of vitamin C deficiency.

Let's dive in.

BUT FIRST: *WHAT IS VITAMIN C?*

Vitamin C, also known as ascorbic acid, is a nutrient with numerous crucial functions related to human health [1]. The nutrient, along with eight other vitamins, is water-soluble, which means it dissolves in water. Once ingested, your body absorbs vitamin C quickly, shuttling it to different tissues.

Unlike fat-soluble vitamins, such as A, E, and K, the body cannot store excess vitamin C for later use, so we must get enough of the nutrient daily. Excess amounts get excreted through urine and sweat, which means toxicity is rare.

FIVE INCREDIBLE BENEFITS OF VITAMIN C
1. Strong Immunity

Each day, the immune system defends you against countless invaders that want to make your body their new home. Many of these intruders give up without a fight, but some make it inside and even gain control of your body for a while. A common example of such invaders is viruses.

A big reason why people turn to vitamin C supplements is to strengthen their immune system, especially while dealing with the flu or common cold. While research doesn't suggest that vitamin C can help us overcome the flu or common cold more quickly, a fair amount of data shows that the nutrient is crucial for our immunity [2].

For one, the nutrient promotes white blood cell production [3, 4]. These cells are essential in protecting the body from infections and are the slowest to restore after illness [3]. Similarly, increasing vitamin C levels in the body protects white blood cells from oxidative stress.

Second, research suggests that vitamin C can strengthen the skin's barrier and prevent invaders from entering your body [5]. The nutrient gets transported to the skin, where it acts as an antioxidant.

Interestingly, some research finds that patients with pneumonia are more likely to have low vitamin C levels [6]. Further, vitamin C administration appears to help them overcome the illness more quickly [7].

2. Healthy Iron Levels

Iron is an essential mineral with functions related to oxygen transportation throughout the body [8]. The mineral supports oxygen transportation through hemoglobin to cells. As a result, your cells can produce energy more efficiently, leading to improved cognition, higher energy levels, and overall well-being.

A notable symptom of iron deficiency is anemia—a condition where your body has lower levels of red blood cells [9]. As a result, you experience symptoms like extreme fatigue, muscle weakness, pale skin, brain fog, and more.

Vitamin C is beneficial because it improves iron absorption, reducing the risk of deficiencies. The effect is well pronounced on poorly absorbed iron, such as that coming from many non-meat sources [10]. In other words, healthy vitamin C levels would be beneficial for preventing iron deficiency in people who don't consume that much meat.

In one paper, 65 children with symptoms of anemia were given a vitamin C supplement [11]. Researchers noted marked improvements in symptoms within six weeks.

3. Potentially Lower Risk of Disease

Each day, the body carries numerous metabolic processes that depend on oxygen for energy production [12]. Many of these processes generate reactive oxygen species (ROS)—unstable molecules with essential functions for our health.

The problem is that accumulating too many of these unstable molecules can damage healthy cells and put people at a higher risk of diseases, such as diabetes and cancer [13]. To counteract these adverse effects, the body has antioxidant functions that prevent ROS accumulation and reduce the risk of oxidative stress [14].

Aside from the body's abilities, getting certain nutrients from food and supplements is beneficial for boosting our antioxidant capacity. Vitamin C is one of the unique antioxidants in the body [15]. The nutrient protects healthy cells from oxidative stress, reducing the risk of numerous diseases.

According to some research, a higher vitamin C intake can boost our antioxidant capacity by as much as 30 percent, resulting in a much stronger defense from the adverse effects of oxygen species.

4. Improved Cognition and Brain Health

Cognitive issues can occur at any age, and it's our job to do everything we can to prevent them. One good way to reduce the risk of brain-related problems is to increase vitamin C levels in the body [16].

For one, the nutrient plays essential antioxidant functions in the brain, protecting neurons from oxidative stress [17]. As a result, we think more clearly, our memory improves, and we are at a lower risk of brain fog.

Second, research suggests that vitamin C plays a vital role in brain development, making the nutrient essential for children and adolescents [18]. The same paper notes that children are at high risk of hypovitaminosis C and are therefore more likely to experience symptoms of vitamin C deficiency. More on that below.

5. Optimal Growth and Development

While most people know vitamin C as 'that nutrient for a strong immune system,' its roles within the body are far more nuanced. Another essential function of vitamin C relates to collagen synthesis [19].

Collagen is the most abundant protein in the body and serves a crucial structural role in our bones, muscles, organs, connective tissues, and more [20]. Adequate collagen levels lead to healthy joints, strong muscles, and more. Collagen is also crucial for growth and development, especially in children, because demands for the protein increase as children grow up and enter their teenage years.

Research also notes that having adequate vitamin C levels and producing more collagen promotes wound healing, which is particularly important during childhood [21].

VITAMIN C DOSAGE RECOMMENDATIONS AND SOURCES

The bare minimum vitamin C dose is 10 mg per day, according to research. That amount is enough for most people to avoid scurvy—severe vitamin C deficiency [22]. But, studies also show that the human body needs far more than just 10 mg daily for optimal levels of the nutrient [23].

Most recent guidelines recommend that men get up to 90 mg daily and women - 75 mg. Children and teenagers can remain healthy with slightly less vitamin C each day:

- 0 to 6 months - 40 mg
- 7 months to a year - 50 mg
- 1 to 3 years - 15 mg
- 4 to 8 years - 25 mg
- 9 to 13 years - 45 mg
- 14 to 18 years (females) - 65 mg
- 14 to 18 years (males) - 75 mg

Some of the best vitamin C sources include:

- Cherries - 25 percent daily value per cup
- Kiwi - 278 percent daily value per cup (sliced)
- Oranges - 85 percent daily value per small fruit
- Grapefruit - 52 percent daily value per 100 grams
- Mandarins - 39 percent daily value per medium-sized fruit
- Lemons - 51 percent daily value per small fruit
- Strawberries - 141 percent daily value per cup
- Broccoli - 50 percent daily value per cup
- Kale - 89 percent daily value per cup (raw)
- Tomatoes - 28 percent daily value per one medium-sized fruit
- Bell peppers - 106 percent daily value per cup
- Brussel sprouts - 124 percent daily value per cup

Kiwi is the best vitamin C source, but there are plenty of other foods for children and adults to cover their daily needs.

THE HIDDEN DANGERS OF VITAMIN C DEFICIENCY

According to some research, scurvy is more common in children from developing countries, which is still surprising, given that a mere 10 mg of vitamin C daily prevents the condition [24]. Symptoms often include bleeding gums, chronic fatigue, muscle weakness, pale skin, low mood, severe joint pain, etc.

But, as discussed above, scurvy is not the only thing to worry about, as mild to moderate deficiencies are still relatively common and can lead to symptoms. Two of the most widespread symptoms of early vitamin C deficiency are appetite loss and irritability. Children are also likely to experience gingival issues, such as gum swelling and bleeding. Loss of teeth is also a risk, but it typically results from prolonged and severe deficiency.

More significant vitamin C deficiency, bordering on scurvy, can lead to impaired wound healing, skin problems, and psychological changes [25].

CONCLUSION

While most people see vitamin C as something we should pay attention to during illness, the nutrient has numerous other vital functions. Among its most notable roles, vitamin C is critical for immune system health, cognition, brain development, growth, iron absorption, and longevity.

A vitamin C deficiency can develop over a long period, and most people don't notice symptoms until they become too pronounced to ignore.

Consuming enough vitamin C is necessary for optimal development, brain health, and overall well-being. Plenty of foods, including oranges, kiwi, and bell peppers, are good sources of the nutrient.

Supplementation is also a viable option, especially in the form of a well-formulated multivitamin. Such products provide good amounts of vitamins and minerals, promoting good health and well-being.

REFERENCES

1. www.ncbi.nlm.nih.gov/pmc/articles/PMC4959991/
2. www.ncbi.nlm.nih.gov/pmc/articles/PMC5707683/
3. www.ncbi.nlm.nih.gov/pmc/articles/PMC5874527/
4. www.pubmed.ncbi.nlm.nih.gov/25157026/
5. www.sciencedirect.com/science/article/abs/pii/S0891584998001324
6. www.pubmed.ncbi.nlm.nih.gov/15139458/
7. www.pubmed.ncbi.nlm.nih.gov/23925826/
8. www.ncbi.nlm.nih.gov/pmc/articles/PMC3999603/
9. www.ncbi.nlm.nih.gov/pmc/articles/PMC3685880/
10. www.pubmed.ncbi.nlm.nih.gov/20200263/
11. www.pubmed.ncbi.nlm.nih.gov/1642785/
12. www.pubmed.ncbi.nlm.nih.gov/32352946/
13. www.ncbi.nlm.nih.gov/pmc/articles/PMC5551541/
14. www.ncbi.nlm.nih.gov/pmc/articles/PMC6204759/
15. www.pubmed.ncbi.nlm.nih.gov/12569111/
16. www.ncbi.nlm.nih.gov/pmc/articles/PMC6454201/
17. www.ncbi.nlm.nih.gov/pmc/articles/PMC4691042/
18. www.ncbi.nlm.nih.gov/pmc/articles/PMC8156420/
19. www.pubmed.ncbi.nlm.nih.gov/18505499/
20. www.pubmed.ncbi.nlm.nih.gov/24443018/
21. www.pubmed.ncbi.nlm.nih.gov/34064689/
22. www.ncbi.nlm.nih.gov/books/NBK493187/
23. www.ncbi.nlm.nih.gov/books/NBK499877/
24. www.ncbi.nlm.nih.gov/pmc/articles/PMC4411344/
25. www.ped-rheum.biomedcentral.com/articles/10.1186/s12969-015-0020-1

VITAMIN D

Vitamin D is a nutrient with many essential functions in the body. Unfortunately, deficiencies are relatively common, and symptoms often take time to surface.

Today's chapter will explore this unique nutrient, how it differs from other vitamins, its role in the body, and much more.

Let's dive in and explore.

WHAT IS VITAMIN D?

Despite its name, vitamin D isn't a vitamin but a group of fat-soluble secosteroids (steroid hormones) with varied functions inside the body [1]. Fat-soluble means we can store these compounds in the adipose (fatty) tissue for later use [2].

You might have heard people call vitamin D 'the sunshine vitamin.' It isn't a coincidence because your body produces the hormone from cholesterol when you expose your skin to direct sunlight.

The group of hormones collectively known as vitamin D carries various essential functions in the body and are crucial for bone health, muscle function, and more.

A notable issue with vitamin D is that the primary way of getting the nutrient is by exposing your skin to sunlight, which isn't always possible [1]. For instance, people who spend large chunks of their days indoors or live in colder climates are less likely to soak up enough of the nutrient. On top of that, only a handful of foods provide some vitamin D, making it even more challenging to maintain healthy levels.

The two dietary forms of vitamin D are [1]:

- D2 (ergocalciferol), found in certain plants, yeast, and fungi
- D3 (cholecalciferol), found in some animal products

Of the two, vitamin D3 appears to raise blood concentrations much more effectively than D2.

FOUR UNIQUE BENEFITS OF VITAMIN D
1. Benefits Related to Mental Health

Mental health is a somewhat taboo topic, especially among men. But, regardless of how we feel about it, good mental health is necessary for leading a rich, long, and fulfilling life. According to data, depression and similar conditions are widespread globally and can affect people from all walks of life, including children and teenagers [3].

Learning to manage our mental health begins by recognizing its importance. Studies show that vitamin D levels can impact our mental health and well-being.

According to research, vitamin D could play a vital role in mental health and in the treatment and prevention of depression. In one recent review and meta-analysis, researchers looked at 25 trials and 7,534 participants [4]. Data showed that vitamin D intake of less than 4,000 IU for over eight weeks had notable benefits related to mental health.

In a questionnaire study, researchers examined the relationship between hypovitaminosis D (insufficient vitamin D levels) on mood disorders, quality of life, and other parameters in fibromyalgia patients [5]. Five hundred ninety-three participants were surveyed over 16 months, and slightly more than a fifth suffered from hypovitaminosis D (serum vitamin D levels lower than 25 ng/mL). According to their data, insufficient vitamin D levels were linked to higher anxiety and depression scores among subjects.

A systematic review and meta-analysis from a few years ago pointed out that vitamin D supplementation was effective at reducing symptoms of depression in studies where it improved levels in the body [6].

2. Crucial for Bone Integrity and Health

Vitamin D is often linked to bone health, and rightfully so. According to data, having adequate levels of the nutrient promotes calcium and phosphorus absorption from the gut [7]. Both minerals are essential for bone health, and a deficiency can lead to osteoporosis later in life [8].

Our bones are the primary storage 'area' for calcium. Not getting enough of the mineral (or failing to absorb it from the gut) forces the bones to release stored calcium. The gradual release might not cause issues in the short run, but it can lead to a drop in bone mineral density over time.

Research on vitamin D supplementation in the elderly also suggests that it can reduce the risk of osteoporosis and fractures [9].

3. It Can Lower the Risk of Certain Conditions

Vitamin D might not seem all that important for our health. But, aside from its primary benefits, early research suggests that the nutrient can promote health on several fronts and reduce the risk of:

- **Rheumatoid arthritis (RA).** Research finds a clear link between lower vitamin D levels and a higher likelihood of suffering from RA [10]. The condition is characterized by swelling, stiffness, and joint pain, and typically affects the hands, wrists, knees, and feet.
- **Hypertension and cardiovascular disease.** Lower vitamin D levels have been linked to hypertension (high blood pressure) and an elevated risk of suffering from a stroke or heart attack [11].

- **Certain cancers.** While there are numerous categories and subcategories of cancer, each varying in intensity, progression, and outcomes, data suggests that vitamin D can help. According to some research, adequate vitamin D levels can reduce the risk of developing cancer by as much as 60 percent [12]. Still, we must note that exposing your skin to sunlight for too long can lead to sunburns, which can put you at a higher risk of skin cancer [13].
- **Diabetes.** Perhaps surprisingly, vitamin D appears essential for metabolic health. Data suggests that vitamin D deficiencies predispose individuals to type 1 and 2 diabetes [14].

It's important to note that some of the above are *correlations*. For instance, people with lower vitamin D levels are more likely to suffer from cardiovascular disease. But, that could simply be due to an unhealthy lifestyle that includes a lot of time spent indoors, preventing people from optimizing vitamin D levels or moving enough.

4. Necessary for Immune System Function

The body's immune system works every second of every day, scanning for threats and eradicating invaders looking to make your body their home. Aside from helping you deal with the common cold, the immune system is crucial for your well-being and longevity.

According to data, vitamin D is one of several essential nutrients that promote a healthy immune system [15]. Specifically, the nutrient can modulate the innate and adaptive immune responses. The same paper also notes that a vitamin D deficiency increases the risk of autoimmunity (where the immune system attacks healthy body cells) and susceptibility to infections [15].

VITAMIN D DOSAGE RECOMMENDATIONS AND BEST SOURCES

The recommended daily intake of vitamin D is as follows [16]:

- 0 to 12 months - 400 IU (10 mcg)
- 1 to 70 years - 600 IU (15 mcg)
- 70+ years - 800 IU (20 mcg)

According to some sources, the safe upper limit is 4,000 IU (100 mcg) [17]. But, given that vitamin D is fat-soluble, a high intake can eventually lead to significant saturation. Luckily, toxicity through sun exposure is unlikely because your body regulates its production based on needs and concentrations.

Unfortunately, it's challenging to calculate your daily vitamin D intake, given that sun exposure is the primary way to get it. Some sources suggest revealing enough of your skin to direct sunlight daily would optimize vitamin D levels, but that isn't always an option [18]. For instance, you won't be able to get enough vitamin D from the sun when it's cloudy outside. Plus, your country's climate also matters. A person in Canada is more likely to be deficient than someone living in California simply because of the average yearly temperatures.

Relying on healthy eating doesn't fix the issue fully as only a handful of foods provide some amount of vitamin D. These are:
- Egg yolk - 4 to 5 percent daily value per each
- Mushrooms - up to 17 to 18 percent daily value per cup of some varieties
- Herring - 27 percent daily value per 3.5 ounces
- Salmon - 66 percent daily needs per 3.5 ounces
- Canned tuna - 34 percent daily value per 3.5 ounces
- Fortified cow's milk - 10 to 15 percent of daily needs per cup

THE HIDDEN DANGERS OF A VITAMIN D DEFICIENCY

The problem with vitamin D is that deficiencies are relatively common, and anyone can be at risk, even in developed countries like the United States. According to data, over one billion people worldwide are at least somewhat deficient in the nutrient [19]. For reference, that's almost one in seven people.

Another significant problem with vitamin D deficiencies is that symptoms often take time to develop and waiting for signs could mean it's too late to reverse course [8, 14, 15]. Data also finds that older adults are more likely to be vitamin D deficient [20].

Another issue with vitamin D is that the primary way to see if you're deficient and need supplementation is by having blood work done. Vitamin D stores under 12 ng/mL are considered insufficient, and levels over 20 ng/mL are deemed healthy. Some sources suggest that up to 30 ng/mL is necessary for optimal health [21].

CONCLUSION

Vitamin D can be confusing to understand. Unlike other nutrients, vitamin D isn't an actual vitamin or mineral but a group of hormones your body produces in response to direct sunlight. As such, it can be challenging to determine if you or your children are getting the necessary amount for good health.

Certain foods can raise vitamin D levels, but sometimes supplementation is necessary to keep a deficiency at bay and stay healthy in the long run.

REFERENCES

1. www.ncbi.nlm.nih.gov/pmc/articles/PMC3356951/
2. www.ncbi.nlm.nih.gov/books/NBK534869/
3. www.dbsalliance.org/education/depression/statistics/
4. www.pubmed.ncbi.nlm.nih.gov/32365423/
5. www.pubmed.ncbi.nlm.nih.gov/32022867/
6. www.ncbi.nlm.nih.gov/pmc/articles/PMC4011048/
7. www.pubmed.ncbi.nlm.nih.gov/7015957/
8. www.ncbi.nlm.nih.gov/pmc/articles/PMC4784773/
9. www.pubmed.ncbi.nlm.nih.gov/23320612/
10. www.ncbi.nlm.nih.gov/pmc/articles/PMC3539179/
11. www.pubmed.ncbi.nlm.nih.gov/31172459/
12. www.pubmed.ncbi.nlm.nih.gov/17556697/
13. www.ncbi.nlm.nih.gov/pmc/articles/PMC2873840/
14. www.pubmed.ncbi.nlm.nih.gov/15971062/
15. www.ncbi.nlm.nih.gov/pmc/articles/PMC3166406/
16. www.ods.od.nih.gov/factsheets/VitaminD-HealthProfessional/
17. www.ncbi.nlm.nih.gov/books/NBK56070/
18. www.pubmed.ncbi.nlm.nih.gov/21158934/
19. www.ncbi.nlm.nih.gov/books/NBK532266/
20. www.pubmed.ncbi.nlm.nih.gov/17608242/
21. www.pubmed.ncbi.nlm.nih.gov/18400738/

VITAMIN E

It's no secret that our nutritional choices significantly affect our health, well-being, and longevity. One huge reason is that foods supply the many essential nutrients we need to function at our best, keep disease at bay, and feel great.

This chapter will go over one essential nutrient necessary for many things: vitamin E. More specifically, we'll go over what the nutrient is, how it functions, what benefits it offers, and much more.

Ready? Let's dive in.

WHAT IS VITAMIN E?

Vitamin E is one of 13 essential vitamins your body needs to function normally and carry out many processes that keep you healthy [1, 2]. Along with A, D, and K, vitamin E is fat-soluble, meaning we can store it in adipose (fat) tissue for later use. In contrast, nutrients like vitamin C are water-soluble, and excess amounts are typically excreted through sweat and urine.

Though most people consider vitamin E a single nutrient, the term refers to eight compounds with powerful antioxidant functions in the body. Four are tocopherols (antioxidants with plant origins that protect lipids in the body), and four are tocotrienols (antioxidants with similar functions but a slightly different chemical formula).

The most notable functions of vitamin E relate to immune system function, cell health, and our skin [3, 4]. Like vitamin C, vitamin E possesses potent antioxidant properties, making the nutrient necessary for protecting healthy cells from oxidative stress [1]. Data also links vitamin E with protection against dermatitis and fatty liver disease [5, 6].

Interestingly, exposure to UV and sunlight appears to lower vitamin E levels in the skin, which can lead to issues [7]. Fortunately, a true vitamin E deficiency is rare, and the nutrient is abundant in many foods and skincare products.

FOUR IMPRESSIVE HEALTH BENEFITS OF VITAMIN E
1. Oxidative Protection

Each day, your body carries out numerous metabolic processes. Some are related to your health, and others are necessary for brain function. Most of these internal activities generate reactive oxygen species (ROS)—unstable molecules with some health benefits [8].

Under normal circumstances, these oxygen species don't pose much of a threat because your body has a system for dealing with them. Unfortunately, ROS can accumulate over time and promote oxidative stress, speeding up the aging process and increasing the risk of chronic conditions [9, 10].

Instead of relying on your body to deal with oxidative stress alone, you should support its efforts by consuming enough antioxidants from various foods. Vitamin E is a potent antioxidant that strengthens the body's defenses against damage to healthy cells, reducing the risk of health problems later in life [1].

Research shows that supplementing with vitamin E can strengthen the defense against ROS in specific populations [11]. In one study, participants with diabetic nephropathy (kidney damage due to high blood glucose levels) took 800 IU of vitamin E daily for twelve weeks (source). At the end of the experiment, the subjects had higher glutathione peroxidase (GPx) levels (an antioxidant enzyme) [12].

2. Skin Health

If you're looking for natural ways to improve your skin health, start by taking good care of your vitamin intake. Vitamin E, along with C, D, and other compounds, is necessary for maintaining your skin's elastic properties, making it appear vibrant and more youthful [4, 13].

Despite the limited research so far, early findings have been promising. For example, in one paper from 2021, researchers noted that vitamin E supplementation could be beneficial against eczema—a skin condition characterized by redness and itchiness [5].

Vitamin E is also added to many topical creams and cosmetic products precisely because of its promise as a skin-enhancing nutrient. Among the products containing vitamin E are sunscreens, anti-aging serums, makeup products, and eye creams.

3. Possible Cardiovascular Protection

According to statistics, cardiovascular disease is one of the leading causes of death worldwide [14]. On top of that, heart-related disease leads to disabilities and low quality of life. To make matters worse, children are also not immune to such health issues. Data suggests that one in 100 babies has a congenital heart defect (CHD) [15].

Taking good care of our cardiovascular health is a life-long obligation everyone must take seriously. Good ways to improve cardiovascular outcomes include maintaining a healthy weight, exercising regularly, sleeping well, and managing stress [16, 17].

Nutrition also plays a significant role in the equation, and it appears that vitamin E is necessary for heart health. A systematic review from 2019 suggested that vitamin E supplementation can reduce systolic blood pressure (the pressure in your arteries when your heart beats), possibly leading to better health outcomes [18].

One study suggested that pairing vitamin E with omega-3 fatty acids could lead to a drop in low-density lipoprotein (LDL) cholesterol and blood triglyceride in patients with metabolic syndrome [19]. Research shows that high LDL cholesterol puts us at a higher risk of cardiovascular disease [20].

4. Potential Cognitive Benefits

Good cognition impacts our productivity, determines how well we learn things and retain information, and makes us better problem-solvers. As with most aspects of our health and well-being, our cognitive abilities depend on numerous things, including genetics, mood, excitability, engagement, etc.

According to research, maintaining healthy vitamin E levels is necessary for preventing cognitive decline, especially as we age [21]. One potential mechanism behind these effects could be vitamin E's powerful antioxidant functions. Maintaining healthy levels of the vitamin could protect brain cells from oxidative stress, leading to a healthier and sharper mind.

VITAMIN E DOSAGE RECOMMENDATIONS AND BEST SOURCES

As discussed earlier, vitamin E is a group of eight compounds, each with a unique biological activity in the body. Of the eight, alpha-tocopherol is the only one recognized to meet human needs [22].

The recommended vitamin E daily intake is as follows [22]:

- 0 to 6 months - 4 mg
- 7 to 12 months - 5 mg
- 1 to 3 years - 6 mg

- 4 to 8 years - 7 mg
- 9 to 13 years - 11 mg
- 14+ years - 15 mg

Doses of up to 1,000 mg per day appear safe and well-tolerated in adults [22]. Still, most of the data is from short-term studies on small groups of people. Since vitamin E is fat-soluble and we store excess amounts for later use, you should avoid excessive intakes because that could lead to toxicity.

Here are some excellent food sources and their respective quantity per serving:

- Sunflower seeds - 66 percent of daily needs
- Sunflower oil - 37 percent of daily needs
- Mamey sapote - 39 percent of daily needs
- Wheat germ oil - 130 percent of daily needs
- Peanuts - 16 percent of daily needs
- Avocado - 14 percent of daily needs
- Almonds - 48 percent of daily needs
- Almond oil - 36 percent of daily needs
- Brazil nuts - 11 percent of daily needs
- Hazelnuts - 28 percent of daily needs
- Hazelnut oil - 43 percent of daily needs

THE DANGERS OF A VITAMIN E DEFICIENCY

According to research, vitamin E deficiency is extremely rare in people and is most likely due to an underlying metabolic problem rather than poor nutritional choices [23].

As discussed above, vitamin E is one of four fat-soluble vitamins, and excess amounts are not excreted through sweat or urination but stored for later use. As such, running out of usable vitamin E is highly unlikely.

In any case, the only accurate way to determine your vitamin E status is to have tests done. Symptoms of a deficiency include impaired coordination, poor reflexes, and muscle weakness.

IS THERE A RISK OF VITAMIN E TOXICITY?

Research doesn't indicate any dangers of consuming vitamin E-rich foods, even in high quantities. But, the same cannot be said about supplementation. Most products cover all your daily vitamin E needs, often going overboard. Combining such products with a diet that's moderately rich in vitamin E could result in toxicity. One significant problem with high vitamin E levels is that it could become harder for blood to clot, resulting in severe and potentially life-threatening bleeding.

Vitamin E can also interact with certain medications and create problems. For example, vitamin E supplements can interact with warfarin—a type of drug given to people to prevent blood clots from forming. These effects appear particularly common in people with vitamin K deficiency [24].

People who suspect they might have lower vitamin E levels should consult their doctor and have tests done. Supplementation can be beneficial, but it is important to be supervised by a medical professional and have tests done regularly to ensure levels don't get too high.

CONCLUSION

Vitamin E is one of 26+ essential nutrients your body needs to function. Along with vitamins A, D, and K, vitamin E is fat-soluble, and we can store it in fatty tissue for later use.

Despite being called a vitamin, E isn't a traditional nutrient like, say, vitamin C. Instead, vitamin E refers to a group of eight potent antioxidants that protect the body's cells from reactive oxygen species, reducing the risk of disease. Vitamin E is also necessary for cardiovascular health, immunity, cognition, and lots more.

Luckily for us, plenty of foods are rich in vitamin E, and the actual risk of a deficiency is relatively low.

REFERENCES

1. www.ncbi.nlm.nih.gov/pmc/articles/PMC3997530/
2. www.ncbi.nlm.nih.gov/books/NBK557737/
3. www.ncbi.nlm.nih.gov/pmc/articles/PMC7011499/
4. www.pubmed.ncbi.nlm.nih.gov/27559512/
5. www.pubmed.ncbi.nlm.nih.gov/33070130/
6. www.pubmed.ncbi.nlm.nih.gov/33335561/
7. www.pubmed.ncbi.nlm.nih.gov/18852418/
8. www.ncbi.nlm.nih.gov/pmc/articles/PMC5551541/
9. www.ncbi.nlm.nih.gov/pmc/articles/PMC3101336/
10. www.ncbi.nlm.nih.gov/pmc/articles/PMC5927356/
11. www.pubmed.ncbi.nlm.nih.gov/29891745/
12. www.sciencedirect.com/topics/neuroscience/glutathione-peroxidase
13. www.ncbi.nlm.nih.gov/pmc/articles/PMC7827176/
14. www.cdc.gov/nchs/fastats/leading-causes-of-death.htm
15. www.choa.org/parent-resources/heart/signs-of-heart-problems-in-children-and-teens
16. www.ncbi.nlm.nih.gov/pmc/articles/PMC6557987/
17. www.pubmed.ncbi.nlm.nih.gov/22473079/
18. www.pubmed.ncbi.nlm.nih.gov/30846828/
19. www.pubmed.ncbi.nlm.nih.gov/31405672/
20. www.pubmed.ncbi.nlm.nih.gov/10712410/
21. www.ncbi.nlm.nih.gov/pmc/articles/PMC8625211/
22. www.ods.od.nih.gov/factsheets/VitaminE-HealthProfessional/
23. www.ncbi.nlm.nih.gov/books/NBK519051/
24. www.ncbi.nlm.nih.gov/pmc/articles/PMC5760175/

VITAMIN K

There are over two dozen essential nutrients we need to consume to maintain our health, keep disease at bay, and feel at our best. Some of the most popular ones include calcium, vitamin C, and B complex.

Today's chapter will go over a relatively less known nutrient: vitamin K. But, as you'll see in a moment, the vitamin serves several crucial functions in the body, despite not being as popular as many of its brothers (vitamins) and cousins (minerals).

Let's dive in and explore.

WHAT IS VITAMIN K?

Vitamin K is one of the 26 essential nutrients your body needs to function optimally. The nutrient was discovered almost a century ago in 1929 by Carl Peter Henrik Dam. He discovered the nutrient by chance while running experiments on sterol metabolism [1]. Vitamin K was immediately associated with blood coagulation, and researchers isolated and studied the nutrient in the following decades.

Today, vitamin K isn't as popular as its brothers—vitamins B, C, and D, to name a few. Still, the nutrient is crucial for our health, and getting enough of it is necessary for many internal processes.

There are two primary forms of vitamin K [2]:

- Vitamin K1 (phylloquinone) - a form of the nutrient found in plants

- Vitamin K2 (menaquinone) - a form found in animal products and fermented foods

Like vitamins A and E, K2 is a collection of compounds with essential bodily functions. Two of the most important forms are MK-4 (menatetrenone) and MK-7 (menaquinone-7).

WHAT BENEFITS DOES VITAMIN K PROVIDE?

1. Vitamin K May Promote Bone Health

Bone health isn't a topic most people discuss, but our bones provide structure, hold our muscles, and allow us to move. Our bones also protect crucial organs, like the brain, heart, and lungs. On top of that, our bones store large amounts of two essential minerals: calcium and potassium. These nutrients contribute to bone strength, and the body can use small amounts of the minerals during periods of low dietary intake.

Most people don't think about bone health because problems take a long time to develop, often decades. By the time symptoms surface, problems are much more challenging to fix. For instance, osteoporosis is characterized by weak and fragile bones, but people are typically diagnosed after experiencing a fracture [3].

Vitamin K is necessary for bone health because it plays an integral role in calcium metabolism. Specifically, vitamin K2 activates osteocalcin and matrix GLA—two proteins with calcium-binding properties that play an important role in bone formation [4, 5].

Studies find that vitamin K offers significant benefits for bone health in different populations [6, 7]. In fact, vitamin K2 supplements have been approved as part of treatment for osteoporosis in Japan since 1995 [8].

2. It Could Promote Dental Health

Vitamin K plays a crucial role in bone metabolism, so it isn't unreasonable to assume that the nutrient promotes dental health. Unfortunately, no human studies have established the connection, so we must look at data from animal trials.

Osteocalcin, a protein we mentioned earlier, is crucial for dental health, and data shows that vitamin K2 activates it [4, 5]. Regarding dental health, osteocalcin appears to trigger the formation of dentin—a yellowish tissue that makes up the bulk of our teeth [9, 10].

3. The Nutrient Is Necessary for Cardiovascular Health

Statistics show that cardiovascular disease is the leading cause of death and disability. One reason a person might develop cardiovascular issues is due to calcium build-up inside the arteries surrounding the heart [11, 12].

Vitamin K could offer heart-related benefits because it may prevent the build-up of calcium in the arteries. In one study, 4807 subjects were followed for seven to ten years, and researchers looked at the link between vitamin K2 intake and risk of cardiovascular disease [13]. Data suggested that a higher vitamin K intake was associated with a reduced risk of cardiovascular disease, all-cause mortality, and aortic atherosclerosis (plaque build-up in the aorta).

A review of existing data had similar findings [14]. Researchers looked at previous studies with over 16000 women and found that a higher vitamin K2 intake is correlated with a reduced risk of cardiovascular disease. Interestingly, vitamin K1 wasn't shown to be beneficial for cardiovascular health.

4. Vitamin K Has Cancer-Fighting Properties

According to data, cancer is the second leading cause of mortality worldwide, coming only after cardiovascular disease [15]. The collection of diseases accounts for over 600,000 global deaths each year.

Despite the advancements in modern medicine, cancer is still tricky to manage, even if it gets diagnosed in the early stages. There are numerous forms of the disease, each with its unique risks, progression rate, and more.

Interestingly, some data suggests that vitamin K2 could be beneficial for certain forms of cancer and possibly contribute to longer survival times [16, 17].

5. It Is Necessary for Blood Clotting

As discussed earlier in the guide, vitamin K was connected to blood coagulation quickly after its discovery [1]. Specifically, vitamin K plays a vital role in the production of proteins needed for blood clotting. One example of such protein is prothrombin—a compound produced in the liver that works with other clotting factors to promote coagulation.

HOW MUCH VITAMIN K DO YOU NEED (AND WHAT ARE SOME GOOD SOURCES)?

According to guidelines, adults need roughly one microgram (mcg; 0.001 milligrams) of vitamin K per kilogram [18]. So, if we take a 55-kilogram woman, she should consume up to 65 mcg of the nutrient daily.

According to the Institute of Medicine, children and teenagers might need slightly larger amounts of the nutrient each day [19]:

- 0 to 6 months - 2 mcg
- 7 to 12 months - 2.5 mcg
- 1 to 3 years - 30 mcg
- 4 to 8 years - 55 mcg
- 9 to 13 years - 60 mcg
- 14 to 18 years - 75 mcg

Numerous foods are rich in vitamin K, but most appear to provide the less active K1. Your body can convert K1 to the more potent K2 form, but the process is inefficient, so it's vital to pick more foods rich in the more active K2 instead of relying on conversion [20].

We've outlined several good sources with their respective quantities per serving:

- Swiss chard - 300+ percent daily needs
- Collard greens - 300+ percent daily needs
- Spinach - 121 percent daily needs
- Kale - 400+ percent daily needs
- Broccoli - 92 percent daily needs
- Mustard greens - 300+ percent daily needs
- Green beans - 17 to 25 percent daily needs
- Brussel sprouts - 90 percent daily needs
- Kiwi - 23 percent daily needs
- Chicken - 43 percent daily needs
- Organ meat - 50 to 60 percent daily needs
- Pork - 45 percent daily needs
- Cheese - 15 to 20 percent daily needs

Green vegetables offer large amounts of the nutrient, but animal products are also valuable for getting enough of the active K2 form.

IS THERE A RISK OF VITAMIN K DEFICIENCY (AND WHAT CAN YOU DO ABOUT IT)?

The risk of a vitamin K deficiency is quite low, given that many foods include at least small quantities of the nutrient. Even if a person mostly consumes vitamin K1, the body can convert some amount of it into the more active K2 form [20].

Vitamin K deficiency appears most prominently in infants, and it is called vitamin K deficiency bleeding (VKDB) [21]. The condition is characterized by excessive bleeding in infants that don't have enough vitamin K to form blood clots. External bleeding is more noticeable and easier to treat, but there is also a risk of internal bleeding that can be difficult to see.

Some sources recommend newborn babies receive a vitamin K shot to raise blood levels immediately. Part of the vitamin K is absorbed by the body and released steadily over several months, ensuring babies have enough of the nutrient to avoid a deficiency.

ARE VITAMIN K TOXICITIES COMMON, AND WHAT SHOULD YOU DO ABOUT THEM?

Like many other essential nutrients, vitamin K toxicity is rare [2]. A natural organic compound called menadione appears to be the only substance capable of causing vitamin K toxicity. Luckily, menadione has no use for us.

There are no recorded cases of toxicity from K1 and K2 intake, and there isn't an upper intake level (UL) [2].

CONCLUSION

Vitamin K is one of four fat-soluble nutrients (along with vitamins A, D, and E). The nutrient was discovered by accident but was instantly linked to blood coagulation—an essential bodily process that keeps us from bleeding out.

Aside from blood coagulation, vitamin K protects the body against certain cancers and cardiovascular disease, promotes bone and dental health, and more.

The two primary forms of the vitamin are K1 (phylloquinone), primarily found in plants, and K2 (menaquinone), found in animal products. Vitamin K2 is a collection of compounds with various essential bodily functions.

A vitamin K deficiency is unlikely because most foods contain at least some amount of the nutrient. The body can convert vitamin K1 to K2, though the process appears inefficient, so it's best to include some animal products in your diet.

REFERENCES

1. www.pubmed.ncbi.nlm.nih.gov/23183291/
2. www.ncbi.nlm.nih.gov/books/NBK551578/
3. www.ncbi.nlm.nih.gov/books/NBK441901/
4. www.ncbi.nlm.nih.gov/pmc/articles/PMC7399911/
5. www.ncbi.nlm.nih.gov/books/NBK536983/
6. www.pubmed.ncbi.nlm.nih.gov/16801507/
7. www.pubmed.ncbi.nlm.nih.gov/23525894/
8. www.pubmed.ncbi.nlm.nih.gov/18830045/
9. www.pubmed.ncbi.nlm.nih.gov/11856645/
10. www.ncbi.nlm.nih.gov/pmc/articles/PMC6214857/
11. www.ahajournals.org/doi/10.1161/jaha.116.003815
12. www.pubmed.ncbi.nlm.nih.gov/23529983/
13. www.pubmed.ncbi.nlm.nih.gov/15514282/
14. www.pubmed.ncbi.nlm.nih.gov/19179058/
15. www.cdc.gov/nchs/fastats/leading-causes-of-death.htm
16. www.pubmed.ncbi.nlm.nih.gov/16400650/
17. www.ncbi.nlm.nih.gov/pmc/articles/PMC5958717/
18. www.nhs.uk/conditions/vitamins-and-minerals/vitamin-k/
19. www.ods.od.nih.gov/Health_Information/Dietary_Reference_Intakes.aspx
20. www.ncbi.nlm.nih.gov/pmc/articles/PMC7353270/
21. www.ncbi.nlm.nih.gov/books/NBK536983/

CALCIUM

We've all heard of calcium—the nutrient most people associate with bone health. While that is one of calcium's functions in the body, it is far from the only benefit.

Today's chapter will cover calcium, what it is, what functions it has, what the optimal dose is, and much more.

Let's dive in.

WHAT IS CALCIUM?

Calcium is one of the thirteen essential minerals your body needs to remain healthy and carry out numerous processes [1]. The mineral is most often associated with bone and teeth health, but its functions are far more nuanced than people imagine.

According to research, roughly 99 percent of calcium gets stored in the bones and teeth [2]. The remaining one percent travels in the bloodstream, sending nerve signals, regulating muscle contractions, releasing hormones, and more.

The mineral is crucial for your health, and not getting enough of it forces your body to release calcium from bones and teeth to meet its needs. Unfortunately, doing so weakens your bone integrity and increases the risk of osteoporosis [3].

Like most vitamins and minerals, calcium dissolves in water. Excess amounts of the mineral get excreted through urine to prevent hypercalcemia—dangerously high calcium levels. Because of that, you must get enough calcium from foods every day.

WHAT FUNCTIONS DOES CALCIUM HAVE IN THE BODY?

1. Calcium is Necessary for Nerve Signalling

Calcium is described as the ultimate multitasker in neuron cells due to its many essential functions [4]. Most notably, the mineral supports electrical signals down axons (the thin fiber that runs out of the neuron and carries electrical signals to other nerve cells).

Aside from that, calcium is necessary for muscle contractions. Once your brain commends a muscle to contract, calcium triggers the shortening of muscle fibers by reacting with regulatory proteins [5].

Low calcium levels can lead to tetany—the involuntary contraction of muscles in your body.

2. The Mineral Can Have Beneficial Effects on Metabolic Health

Metabolic disorders like type 2 diabetes are an emerging health threat. According to data, such disorders can increase the risk of cardiovascular disease, stroke, and more [6].

Globally, the prevalence of diabetes was 8.8 percent (415 million) in 2015 and is expected to grow to 10.4 percent (640 million) by 2040 [7]. Further, metabolic syndrome (a cluster of conditions that occur together) appears to be three times more prevalent than diabetes, suggesting that over 1.2 billion people are affected.

The good news is that calcium shows promise in the battle against metabolic disease. A review of human studies noted that adequate calcium intake correlates with a lower risk of metabolic disease [8].

3. It Is Crucial for Bone and Teeth Health

One of calcium's most notable functions in the body relates to bone and teeth health [9]. These tissues serve as a reservoir for the nutrient, and not getting enough of it can cause your bones and teeth to release some into the bloodstream.

Low calcium intake can weaken your bones to the point where they become fragile and take much longer to heal. The condition is known as osteoporosis and is typically diagnosed after a fracture [10].

4. Calcium Can Reduce the Risk of Colon Cancer

Colorectal cancer is the third leading cause of cancer-related death among men and women [11]. Data suggests that the form of cancer is expected to cause over 52,000 deaths in 2022.

The overall risk of lifetime colon cancer is 4.3 percent for men and 4.0 percent for women. Still, factors like genetic predisposition, poor nutrition, and lack of exercise can increase the risk in many people.

Interestingly, research suggests that calcium could play a role in preventing colon cancer. A review of ten studies with over 534,000 participants indicated that a higher calcium intake could reduce the risk of colorectal cancer [12].

A large observational study also found that adequate calcium intake from supplements and dairy can reduce the risk of certain cancers, including that of the colon [13].

5. Potential Benefits During Pregnancy

Pregnant women are at risk of developing preeclampsia—a serious condition characterized by blood pressure elevation, swelling of the limbs, and protein in the urine [14]. The condition typically develops after the 20th week of pregnancy, but it can also occur after the delivery, a condition called postpartum preeclampsia.

According to research, calcium supplementation during pregnancy can reduce the risk of the condition and premature birth. The World Health Organization now recommends calcium supplementation during pregnancy [15].

HOW MUCH CALCIUM SHOULD YOU GET (AND WHAT ARE SOME GOOD SOURCES)?

Like with most other essential nutrients, calcium needs vary by age. Here are the recommended daily intakes based on age [16]:
- 0 to 6 months - 200 mg
- 7 to 12 months - 260 mg
- 1 to 3 years - 700 mg
- 4 to 8 years - 1,000 mg
- 9 to 18 years - 1,300 mg
- 19 to 50 years - 1,000 mg
- 51 to 70 years - 1,200 mg (women); 1,000 mg men
- 70+ years - 1,200 mg

Here are some of the best food sources of calcium with their respective quantities as a percentage of the recommended daily intake (RDI):
- Tofu - 122 percent of daily needs per cup
- Fortified cereal - up to 100 percent of daily needs per serving (depending on the brand)
- Milk - 30 to 35 percent of daily needs per cup
- Yogurt - 25 percent of daily needs per cup
- Sardines - 24 percent of daily needs per three ounces
- Cheese - 24 percent of daily needs per ounce
- Leafy greens - 20 to 25 percent of daily needs per cup
- Almonds - 8 percent of daily needs per ounce
- Seeds - 7 to 11 percent of daily needs per tablespoon

It's important to note that your body needs time to absorb calcium, so it's best to spread your intake over at least two meals and a snack.

Only taking a supplement could theoretically provide enough daily calcium, but you might still end up deficient if you don't absorb it effectively.

Whey and casein protein powders are also good calcium sources. The two types of protein are dairy-based and provide 15 to 50 percent of your daily calcium needs per scoop, depending on the brand.

IS TOO MUCH CALCIUM DANGEROUS?

Calcium is a water-soluble nutrient, but there is a risk of adverse effects if you ingest too much, especially in supplement form. Some early symptoms of excessive calcium consumption include gas, bloating, and constipation.

People who consume large amounts of the nutrient could also be at a higher risk of kidney stones. In one paper, postmenopausal women taking 1,000 mg of calcium daily were at a higher risk of kidney stones [17].

In one review, researchers looked at the existing literature on calcium supplementation and health [18]. The authors focused on previous findings that supplementation increases the risk of myocardial infarction (heart attack).

Their findings were mixed. Some studies found a small or non-existent increase in cardiovascular issues in people supplementing with calcium. For instance, one of the studies suggested that calcium supplements could increase the risk of a heart attack in postmenopausal women [18].

The researchers further suggest there might be cause for concern when routinely consuming 2000 mg or more, but that lower intakes are likely safe [18].

It is likely best to add more calcium-rich foods to your diet instead of resorting to a supplement. Older adults might consider a supplement that offers 500 or fewer milligrams per dose to get the recommended 1,200 mg per day.

CONCLUSION

Calcium is one of the thirteen essential minerals your body needs. The nutrient is necessary for bone health, longevity, muscle contractions, and metabolic health. Oddly enough, some research also suggests that an adequate calcium intake can reduce the risk of colon cancer.

Best practices dictate we should strive to get the mineral through food rather than supplements. Some good options include dairy products, certain nuts, leafy green veggies, tofu, and sardines.

It's best to spread your calcium intake to ensure optimal absorption instead of relying on a single dose of a supplement to cover your needs.

REFERENCES

1. www.ncbi.nlm.nih.gov/books/NBK557683/
2. www.ncbi.nlm.nih.gov/books/NBK56060/
3. www.pubmed.ncbi.nlm.nih.gov/9263260/
4. www.ncbi.nlm.nih.gov/pmc/articles/PMC3249630/
5. www.ncbi.nlm.nih.gov/pmc/articles/PMC1334730/
6. www.cdc.gov/diabetes/basics/type2.html
7. www.ncbi.nlm.nih.gov/pmc/articles/PMC5866840/
8. www.pubmed.ncbi.nlm.nih.gov/33694258/
9. www.ncbi.nlm.nih.gov/pmc/articles/PMC4784773/
10. www.ncbi.nlm.nih.gov/books/NBK441901/
11. www.cancer.org/cancer/colon-rectal-cancer/about/key-statistics.html
12. www.pubmed.ncbi.nlm.nih.gov/15240785/
13. www.pubmed.ncbi.nlm.nih.gov/19237724/
14. www.ncbi.nlm.nih.gov/books/NBK570611/
15. www.ncbi.nlm.nih.gov/pmc/articles/PMC4785477/
16. www.ods.od.nih.gov/factsheets/Calcium-HealthProfessional/
17. www.pubmed.ncbi.nlm.nih.gov/16481635/
18. www.ncbi.nlm.nih.gov/pmc/articles/PMC3257663/

IRON

Iron is a nutrient with a fascinating and complex job: carrying oxygen molecules to all parts of your body.

Of course, iron is crucial for much more than that, and getting enough of it every day is necessary for staying healthy, feeling great, and keeping certain conditions at bay.

Today's guide will show you what iron is, its functions, and how to bump your intake.

Let's review.

WHAT IS IRON?

Iron is one of the 14 essential minerals your body needs to carry out the complex processes that keep you alive and healthy. Along with calcium, potassium, and magnesium, iron is crucial for your health [1].

Most notably, the nutrient is necessary for transporting oxygen throughout the body [1]. All of your body's cells contain iron, but the largest concentrations of the mineral are found in red blood cells.

Your body uses iron to produce hemoglobin—a special protein that carries oxygen molecules [1, 2]. The most common side effect of low iron levels is anemia, a condition characterized by low hemoglobin.

Aside from protecting you against anemia, iron plays a crucial role in energy levels, athletic ability, cognition, and more.

WHAT ARE SOME OF IRON'S CRUCIAL BODILY FUNCTIONS?

1. It Is Essential for Preventing Anemia

As briefly mentioned in the previous point, iron is crucial for preventing anemia—a condition with severe consequences [3]. Anemia can come in many forms depending on the cause.

Iron deficiency anemia is the most common form that results from having too little hemoglobin in red blood cells, as opposed to having too few red blood cells [3]. Your body needs iron to produce hemoglobin, a protein that carries oxygen to all parts of your body.

The issue with anemia is that your body fails to receive the oxygen it needs, and you experience symptoms like:

- Extreme muscle weakness
- Fatigue
- Shortness of breath
- Pale skin
- Brain fog and an inability to concentrate
- Sleepiness
- Dizziness and shakiness
- Cold limbs

What's scary about anemia is that you can experience the symptoms for years and never learn about the cause.

The good news is that consuming enough iron reduces the risk of that form of anemia. It is also an effective treatment for people with iron deficiency anemia. Research suggests that as little as two weeks of iron supplementation can lead to significant improvements [4].

2. Promoting Energy Levels and Well-Being

Fatigue is relatively common and can occur for various reasons [5]. Stress, sleep deprivation, dehydration, and poor diet quality are some risk factors for low energy levels.

Iron can boost your energy levels and promote well-being even if you don't have anemia.

For example, people with lower ferritin could benefit from increasing their iron intake. Ferritin is a protein found in the blood that indicates iron stores.

Women of reproductive age are more likely to benefit from an iron supplement because it can offset the losses from menstruation.

In one study, researchers put together a group of non-anemic women with low ferritin levels who reported feeling fatigued [6]. The women were given 80 mg of elemental iron daily or a placebo for 12 weeks.

Compared to the placebo group, women taking an iron supplement experienced significant improvements in hemoglobin and ferritin levels. They also saw significant improvements in energy levels.

3. Iron Is Important for Cognitive Function

Optimal cognition is necessary for learning, retaining information, recalling things, performing well at work, and leading a more fulfilling life.

Unfortunately, numerous things can get in the way of good cognition. One such example is iron deficiency. Research finds a link between iron levels and cognitive ability in people of all ages [7].

Specifically, when iron levels drop, people often experience an immediate reduction in concentration and the ability to learn.

The good news is that increasing iron levels can reverse these adverse effects, resulting in better cognitive ability and overall concentration [7].

In one randomized control study, 81 girls with non-anemic iron deficiency were randomly given 650 mg of iron twice daily or a placebo for eight weeks [8]. Iron status, test performance, verbal learning, and memory improved in the girls taking iron compared to those given a placebo.

4. The Mineral Is Necessary for Athletic Ability

Iron is crucial for athletic performance on two fronts. First, as discussed earlier, iron is necessary for producing hemoglobin that carries oxygen to all parts of the body, including the brain [1, 2].

Second, iron is vital for producing another protein: myoglobin. The protein is similar to hemoglobin, but it is primarily found in muscle tissue, where it stores oxygen for later use [9].

Getting enough iron is necessary for maintaining healthy levels of myoglobin and supporting your muscles' ability to store oxygen molecules for later use. Having access to oxygen is crucial for your body to produce energy in the form of ATP molecules [10].

The above is especially true for endurance-based activities like cycling and running because they rely heavily on aerobic energy production. Even intense exercise (such as sprinting) heavily depends on oxygen for energy.

5. It Can Help with Restless Leg Syndrome (RLS)

Restless leg syndrome is a medical condition characterized by an uncontrollable urge to move your legs, typically as the result of an uncomfortable feeling.

These feelings typically occur in the evening or at night when you're seated or lying in bed. Moving your limbs brings temporary relief, but the syndrome can disrupt sleep.

While we certainly need more research to conclude, iron appears to be useful against RLS and can alleviate symptoms, leading to better sleep.

In one review paper from 2019, researchers examined the existing literature on the matter. The authors concluded that iron supplementation is associated with improvements in the International Restless Legs Syndrome score in as little as four weeks [11].

HOW MUCH IRON DO YOU NEED (AND WHAT ARE SOME GOOD SOURCES)?

Here are the recommended daily intakes based on age [12]:
- First six months - 0.27 mg
- 7 to 12 months - 11 mg
- 1 to 3 years - 7 mg
- 4 to 8 years - 10 mg
- 9 to 13 years - 8 mg
- 14 to 18 years - 11 mg (boys); 15 mg (girls)
- 19 to 50 years - 8 mg (men); 18 mg (women)
- 50+ years - 8 mg

Pregnant women should consume up to 27 mg of iron daily [12].
Here are some excellent food sources of iron:
- Beef liver - 36 percent of daily needs per 3.5 ounces
- Lentils - 27 percent of daily needs per cup (cooked)
- Beef steak - 20 percent of daily needs per 3.5 ounces
- Dark chocolate - 19 percent of daily needs per ounce
- Shellfish - 17 percent of daily needs per 3.5 ounces
- Quinoa - 16 percent of daily needs per cup (cooked)
- Ground beef - 15 percent of daily needs per 3.5 ounces
- Spinach - 15 percent of daily needs per 3.5 ounces
- Pumpkin seeds - 14 percent of daily needs per ounce
- Dark turkey meat - 8 percent of daily needs per 3.5 ounces
- Broccoli - 6 percent of daily needs per cup

It's important to note that animal products, like red meat, provide heme iron. Heme is a precursor to hemoglobin and is biosynthesized in the liver and bone marrow.

Getting enough heme iron is necessary for optimal absorption and for reducing the risk of deficiency [13]. Vegans and vegetarians are at a higher risk of iron deficiency because plant sources like spinach provide non-heme iron that doesn't get absorbed as effectively [14].

According to research, heme iron can be absorbed as much as four times better than non-heme iron [15].

Aside from people who don't consume animal products, women of childbearing age are at a higher risk of iron deficiency. Menstruation leads to iron loss, so it's beneficial for women to get more of the mineral daily. Supplementation can also be an option.

IS IT POSSIBLE TO GET TOO MUCH IRON IN YOUR DIET?

Healthy people following a balanced diet are not at risk of getting too much iron. The nutrient is water-soluble, and the body readily excretes excess amounts. However, supplementation might be harmful in some cases.

According to data, iron supplements that provide 25 mg or more iron per serving can impair zinc absorption and blood concentrations [16, 17]. A drop in zinc concentration can lead to:
- Gastrointestinal issues
- Hair loss
- Loss of appetite
- Erectile dysfunction
- Irritability and mood swings

Further, a zinc supplement can lead to abdominal cramps, nausea, vomiting, etc. [18, 19]. Taking the supplement with food seems to reduce the risk of such issues.

CONCLUSION

Iron is one of the most important and abundant minerals in the human body. It plays a crucial role in oxygen transportation, and not getting enough can result in iron deficiency anemia that leads to extreme weakness, pale skin, brain fog, and more.

The mineral is also crucial for athletic performance, cognitive function, energy levels, and overall well-being. Some research also suggests that a higher iron intake can help people deal with restless leg syndrome.

It's best to consult your doctor if you suspect you might be deficient or are considering supplementation. Aside from that, you can increase your intake of iron-rich foods: organ and red meat, dark turkey meat, quinoa, dark chocolate, and more.

REFERENCES

1. www.ncbi.nlm.nih.gov/pmc/articles/PMC3999603/
2. www.ncbi.nlm.nih.gov/pmc/articles/PMC7370311/
3. www.ncbi.nlm.nih.gov/books/NBK448065/
4. www.ncbi.nlm.nih.gov/books/NBK448065/
5. www.pubmed.ncbi.nlm.nih.gov/19035066/
6. www.ncbi.nlm.nih.gov/pmc/articles/PMC3414597/
7. www.ncbi.nlm.nih.gov/pmc/articles/PMC4235202/
8. www.pubmed.ncbi.nlm.nih.gov/8855856/
9. www.ncbi.nlm.nih.gov/books/NBK544256/
10. www.ncbi.nlm.nih.gov/pmc/articles/PMC6116100/
11. www.pubmed.ncbi.nlm.nih.gov/30798983/
12. www.ods.od.nih.gov/factsheets/Iron-HealthProfessional/
13. www.ncbi.nlm.nih.gov/books/NBK448204/
14. www.ncbi.nlm.nih.gov/pmc/articles/PMC6367879/
15. www.pubmed.ncbi.nlm.nih.gov/3290310/
16. www.pubmed.ncbi.nlm.nih.gov/9701159/
17. www.pubmed.ncbi.nlm.nih.gov/3522825/
18. www.pubmed.ncbi.nlm.nih.gov/26157809
19. www.pubmed.ncbi.nlm.nih.gov/32468501

MAGNESIUM

From its essential functions in hundreds of biological processes to mental health and blood sugar control, magnesium is crucial for human health.

Today's guide will explore magnesium, what it is, and what effects it has. We will also go over some of the best food sources and the dangers of not consuming enough magnesium.

Let's discuss.

WHAT IS MAGNESIUM?

Magnesium is an essential mineral your body needs to remain healthy [1]. Like all other minerals and most vitamins, magnesium is water-soluble. Your body uses what it needs, and excess amounts get excreted through urine.

The risk of magnesium toxicity is low, but you must get enough of the nutrient through food or supplements every day to avoid a deficiency.

Despite its status as a micronutrient, magnesium plays a crucial role in various bodily systems, processes, and organs. Most notably, the mineral is necessary for brain and heart health, sleep, metabolic functions, mental health, and more.

Magnesium is widely available in many foods (which we will outline below), and you can get the mineral in supplement form.

WHAT ARE SOME OF MAGNESIUM'S FUNCTIONS IN YOUR BODY?

1. Involved in Countless Bodily Processes

Did you know that every cell in your body contains trace amounts of magnesium? The mineral is crucial for many cell functions and getting enough of it allows your body to carry out many processes. Almost half of the magnesium in your body is found in muscles, fluids, organs, and soft tissue [2].

The primary way in which magnesium works is as a cofactor. In other words, the mineral works as a helping molecule, allowing enzymes to carry out hundreds of reactions in your body every day [3].

Some of its most notable functions relate to [3]:

- Regulating various neurotransmitters necessary for sending signals throughout the body
- Muscle contractions
- Creating and repairing DNA and RNA
- Forming new proteins your body needs from the amino acids you ingest through food

2. Potential Benefits for Mental Health

Depression, anxiety, and other issues are becoming more prevalent each year. According to data, up to a fifth of US adults (nearly 50 million people) are suffering from mental illness today [4].

Mental health is a vastly nuanced field, and various factors can increase the risk of depression, anxiety, and similar issues. Such, for example, are leading a sedentary lifestyle, dealing with chronic stress, and losing a loved one [5].

Your nutrition also plays a role in mental health, as data suggests that not getting enough magnesium can increase the risk of depression [6].

Further, supplementation with the mineral can alleviate depressive symptoms in some individuals [7]. The effects appear to be most pronounced in people with a magnesium deficiency.

Interestingly, one paper suggested that magnesium supplementation could alleviate depression regardless of the nutritional status of participants [8].

3. Necessary for Cardiovascular Health

Cardiovascular disease is the leading cause of death worldwide. According to statistics, heart-related problems account for roughly 700,000 deaths in the US yearly [9]. That comes out to a death every 34 seconds.

Magnesium is one of several minerals with a crucial role in cardiovascular health. The nutrient promotes heart health on a couple of big fronts.

First, magnesium is necessary for regulating blood pressure.

High blood pressure (hypertension) is often called the silent killer because it doesn't always bring symptoms, but the arterial pressure can increase the risk of a cardiac event. According to statistics, nearly half of adults in the US have hypertension [10]. Research suggests that a magnesium supplement can reduce blood pressure [11].

Second, magnesium can improve levels of blood triglycerides and cholesterol. High triglycerides and LDL cholesterol levels are linked to atherosclerosis—the narrowing of arteries due to plaque build-up [12]. These effects appear to be particularly pronounced in people with a magnesium deficiency.

4. Could Reduce the Risk of Type 2 Diabetes

Diabetes is a life-long condition characterized by an inability of the body to control its blood sugar levels. The condition typically occurs because the beta cells in the pancreas become damaged and cannot produce, store, and release insulin when the body needs it.

According to statistics, over 37 million Americans (11.3 percent of the population) had diabetes in 2019 [13].

The best way to reduce the risk of type 2 diabetes is to lead a healthier lifestyle [14]. Exercise often, eat a nutritious diet, get enough sleep, and maintain a healthy weight. Getting enough magnesium also appears necessary for managing blood sugar levels.

Data suggests that nearly half of all people with diabetes have low magnesium levels [15]. Further, research indicates that consuming more magnesium reduces the risk of type 2 diabetes [16].

One 2016 systematic review suggests magnesium supplementation improves blood sugar levels and insulin sensitivity in people at risk of diabetes [17].

5. Anti-Inflammatory Effects

Chronic inflammation is an immune system response that continues long after you've dealt with an infection or injury. Like hypertension, chronic inflammation can be dangerous because most people don't realize they have it until the damage has been done.

A low magnesium intake appears to be a risk factor for inflammation and can contribute to faster aging and chronic disease [18].

The good news is that boosting your magnesium intake can have the opposite effect: reduced inflammation. In one review of existing literature, researchers found that magnesium supplementation was correlated with lower levels of certain inflammatory markers [19].

6. It Could Support Your Sleep

According to most guidelines, we should get at least seven hours of sleep per night. Anything less than that can put us in a state of sleep deprivation, making us more likely to experience mood swings, brain fog, and similar.

As discussed earlier, magnesium is involved in hundreds of biological processes. Some of these processes relate to neurotransmitter regulation. One such neurotransmitter is gamma-aminobutyric acid (GABA). It plays a vital role in relaxing the mind and making it easier to fall asleep.

Research also supports the use of magnesium for good sleep. In one study with over 3,900 subjects, magnesium supplementation was linked to better sleep quality and duration [20].

7. Potentially Helpful Against Migraines

Migraine headaches come in the form of throbbing pain on one side of the head. These headaches can vary from mild to debilitating and bring other symptoms like nausea and vomiting [21].

Children can also experience migraine headaches, with up to 11 percent of elementary school-aged children experiencing them occasionally [22].

Some researchers suggest migraines are more likely to occur in people with a magnesium deficiency [23]. Data also shows that magnesium supplementation can reduce the occurrence of migraines and treat them [24].

HOW MUCH MAGNESIUM DO WE NEED (AND IS THERE A RISK OF DEFICIENCY)?

Here are the recommended magnesium daily intakes based on age [25]:

- First 6 months - 30 mg
- 7 to 12 months - 75 mg
- 1 to 3 years - 80 mg
- 4 to 8 years - 130 mg
- 9 to 13 years - 240 mg
- 14 to 18 years (boys) - 410 mg
- 14 to 18 years (girls) - 360 mg
- Adult men - 400 to 420 mg

- Adult women - 310 to 320 mg
- Pregnant women - 350 to 360 mg

Now that we've gone over the recommended intakes, here is a list of some magnesium-rich foods you should add to your diet:

- Spinach - 39 percent of daily needs per cooked cup
- Pumpkin seeds - 37 percent of daily needs per ounce
- Cooked black beans - 30 percent of daily needs per cup
- Cashews - 20 percent of daily needs per ounce
- Dark chocolate - 16 percent of daily needs per ounce
- Avocado - 15 percent of daily needs per medium avocado
- Tofu - 13 percent of daily needs per 3.5 ounces
- Banana - 9 percent of daily needs per large banana
- Salmon - 7 percent of daily needs per 3 ounces

Getting too little magnesium doesn't bring any side effects initially. The kidneys possess the unique function of retaining magnesium during periods of lower intake. Unfortunately, not getting enough magnesium will eventually catch up to you, resulting in a deficiency [25].

Symptoms of a magnesium deficiency include appetite loss, muscle weakness, nausea, shaking, feeling 'pins and needles,' muscle spasms, and more. Older people and those with type 2 diabetes or gastrointestinal issues are more likely to have a magnesium deficiency [25].

IS MAGNESIUM TOXICITY REAL, AND SHOULD WE WORRY ABOUT IT?

Magnesium toxicity is real but highly unlikely because the body readily excretes excess amounts. Even supplementation isn't likely to result in toxicity because most products on the market don't provide such large amounts of the mineral.

Magnesium-rich laxatives and antacids (drugs for indigestion and heartburn) sometimes contain high doses of the mineral and are associated with toxicity [26].

Some common symptoms of magnesium toxicity include low blood pressure, urine retention, hot flashes, arrhythmia (abnormal heartbeat), and, in extreme cases, cardiac arrest.

FINAL WORDS

Magnesium is one of many essential nutrients your body needs to carry out biological processes and stay alive. Some of the mineral's most notable functions relate to energy metabolism, nerve signalling, the production and repair of DNA and RNA, mental health, and protection against chronic inflammation.

Eating a variety of magnesium-rich foods is a great way to get enough of the mineral and prevent a deficiency. Supplementation can also be helpful, given the low toxicity risk, even at higher doses.

REFERENCES

1. www.ncbi.nlm.nih.gov/pmc/articles/PMC5926493/
2. www.mdpi.com/2072-6643/7/9/5388
3. www.pubmed.ncbi.nlm.nih.gov/25540137/
4. www.mhanational.org/issues/2022/mental-health-america-adult-data
5. www.pubmed.ncbi.nlm.nih.gov/19496077/
6. www.pubmed.ncbi.nlm.nih.gov/25748766/
7. www.pubmed.ncbi.nlm.nih.gov/28241991/
8. www.pubmed.ncbi.nlm.nih.gov/28654669/
9. www.cdc.gov/heartdisease/facts.htm
10. www.cdc.gov/bloodpressure/facts.htm
11. www.pubmed.ncbi.nlm.nih.gov/27402922/
12. www.pubmed.ncbi.nlm.nih.gov/28150351/
13. www.diabetes.org/about-us/statistics/about-diabetes
14. www.ncbi.nlm.nih.gov/pmc/articles/PMC6125024/
15. www.pubmed.ncbi.nlm.nih.gov/26322160/
16. www.pubmed.ncbi.nlm.nih.gov/28978672/
17. www.pubmed.ncbi.nlm.nih.gov/27530471/
18. www.pubmed.ncbi.nlm.nih.gov/29403302/
19. www.pubmed.ncbi.nlm.nih.gov/28545353/
20. www.pubmed.ncbi.nlm.nih.gov/34883514/
21. www.ncbi.nlm.nih.gov/books/NBK560787/
22. www.my.clevelandclinic.org/health/diseases/9637-migraines-in-children-and-adolescents
23. www.pubmed.ncbi.nlm.nih.gov/31691193/
24. www.pubmed.ncbi.nlm.nih.gov/29131326/
25. www.ods.od.nih.gov/factsheets/Magnesium-Consumer
26. www.pubmed.ncbi.nlm.nih.gov/17726419/

POTASSIUM

We all know that good nutrition is vital for health, well-being, energy levels, and cognition.

Eating whole and nutritious foods is necessary to supply your body with the nutrients it needs to carry out its many complex processes that sustain life.

One such nutrient we need to consume is potassium. Today's chapter will teach you everything you need to know about potassium, what it is, what functions it has, and lots more.

WHAT IS POTASSIUM?

Potassium is one of the 14 essential minerals your body needs [1]. Like other minerals and most vitamins, potassium is water-soluble (dissolves in water). Your body uses what it needs and excretes excess amounts through urine and sweat.

Your body cannot produce potassium from other nutrients, so it is crucial to get enough of the nutrient through food or supplements every day. Not getting enough potassium can lead to several health issues, which we will discuss later.

The mineral also possesses unique properties and is classified as an electrolyte: an electrically charged molecule (ion) that releases a charge when it dissolves in a fluid [1]. Potassium can conduct electrical impulses throughout the body and regulate certain essential activities.

These electrical signals are necessary for various life-sustaining processes related to the brain, heart, muscles, and more. Some of potassium's special functions relate to nerve transmissions, fluid balance, blood pressure regulation, and muscle contractions.

WHAT ARE POTASSIUM'S FUNCTIONS IN YOUR BODY?

1. Necessary for Nerve Function

The central nervous system (CNS) consists of the brain and spinal cord [2]. It sends and receives messages, making it possible for all body parts to communicate with one another.

For these messages to travel and reach their destination, your body needs assistance from electrolytes.

The messages sent and received by the CNS come in the form of nerve impulses. These impulses regulate various bodily activities, including muscle contractions and heartbeat [2].

Sodium ions are necessary for generating nerve impulses that travel into cells. In contrast, impulses that travel out of cells are generated by potassium ions [3].

Lower potassium levels can prevent the body from effectively producing impulses, impairing nerve function.

2. Contributes to Fluid Balance

Fluid balance refers to two primary things:
- The balance of total fluid your body must maintain to operate at peak efficiency
- The balance between the intracellular and extracellular fluid

The adult human body consists of approximately 60 percent water [4]. Almost half of the water is found in your body's cells and is called intracellular fluid. The remaining water is located outside your cells and is called extracellular fluid.

For your body to maintain a healthy fluid balance, you must get enough sodium and potassium.

Sodium is the primary electrolyte in extracellular fluid and regulates the amount of water your body holds outside its cells. In contrast, potassium is the main player in intracellular fluid and determines how much water your cells contain.

The primary objective is for there to be a roughly equal number of electrolytes inside and outside your cells.

3. Essential For Muscle Contractions

Muscle contractions are straightforward enough. Your brain sends a signal, and your muscles obey.

Unfortunately, the relationship between the mind and muscles is a bit more complex, and optimal muscle function relies on several things. One of these factors is potassium levels in the body.

As discussed above, potassium is necessary for optimal nerve function [1, 3]. Not getting enough of the mineral can impair nerve signalling, leading to weaker muscle contractions.

Of course, potassium is vital for more than flexing your biceps in front of the mirror after a good workout. The mineral is necessary for the heartbeat, and having too much or too little can result in an abnormal heart rhythm (arrhythmia) [5, 6].

4. It Could Regulate Blood Pressure

High blood pressure (hypertension) is a considerable risk factor for cardiovascular disease and early death. According to data, nearly half of the adults in the US suffer from hypertension and could be at a higher risk of cardiovascular disease, heart attack, and more [7].

Consuming enough potassium can have a regulatory impact on your blood pressure and prevent it from increasing too much. As discussed above, potassium is closely related to another mineral and electrolyte: sodium.

One of potassium's functions is to help your body flush out excess sodium, which can otherwise contribute to hypertension. Some research suggests that increasing potassium intake can reduce blood pressure [8].

5. Potential Benefits Against Osteoporosis

Osteoporosis is a condition characterized by fragile bones. The disease often takes decades to develop, and most people get diagnosed after suffering a fracture [9].

Two nutrients necessary for bone health and the prevention of osteoporosis are calcium and vitamin D. According to research, getting more potassium can promote bone health by reducing the amount of calcium the body loses through urine [10].

Additionally, some research finds a correlation between higher potassium intake and bone mass [11].

6. Important for Preventing Kidney Stones

Kidney stones, also known as renal calculi, are hard formations consisting of minerals and salts that form inside the kidneys [12]. The result is a pain in the kidneys, stomach, and groin. Many people also experience a fever, blood in the urine, nausea, and vomiting.

Several factors can increase the risk of kidney stones, including excess body weight, taking certain medications, and not drinking enough water.

As discussed in the previous point, potassium can control how much calcium the body excretes through urine. Getting enough potassium can reduce the amount of calcium passing through the kidneys, leading to a lower risk of kidney formations that turn into stones [13].

HOW MUCH POTASSIUM DO YOU NEED (AND WHAT ARE SOME GOOD SOURCES)?

Here are the recommended potassium daily intakes based on age [14]:
- First 6 months - 400 mg
- 7 to 12 months - 860 mg
- 1 to 3 years - 2,000 mg
- 4 to 8 years - 2,300 mg
- 9 to 13 years - 2,300-2,500 mg
- 14 to 18 years - 2,300 mg (girls); 3,000 mg (boys)
- 19+ years - 2,600 mg (women); 3,400 mg (men)
- Pregnant and breastfeeding - 2,500-2,900 mg

Here are some food sources of potassium and their respective amounts:
- Peanuts - 23 percent of daily needs per cup
- White beans - 21 percent of daily needs per cup
- Yams - 19 percent of daily needs per cup (cooked)
- Soybeans - 19 percent of daily needs per cup
- Sweet potato - 16 percent of daily needs per cup
- Lentils - 15 percent of daily needs per cup
- Avocado - 15 percent of daily needs per large avocado
- Watermelon - 14 percent of daily needs per two wedges
- Coconut water - 13 percent of daily needs per cup
- Potato - 12-14 percent of daily needs cooked potato
- Spinach - 12 percent of daily needs per cup (frozen)
- Butternut squash - 12 percent of daily needs per cup
- Salmon - 11 percent of daily needs per 3 ounces
- Beets - 11 percent of daily needs per cup (boiled)
- Chickpeas - 10 percent of daily needs per cup

- Tuna - 9 percent of daily needs per 3 ounces
- Cod fish - 7 percent of daily needs per 3 ounces

A potassium deficiency (hypokalemia) is unlikely, and most cases are mild. One likely explanation is that covering at least some of their daily needs comes naturally for most people, given how many foods contain the mineral.

Still, you should make an effort to eat a balanced diet and have at least some potassium-rich foods:

- Avocado with your eggs
- A handful of peanuts as an afternoon snack
- Watermelon slices on hot summer days
- Fish for dinner a few days per week

CAN YOU GET TOO MUCH POTASSIUM THROUGH FOOD AND SUPPLEMENTS?

Consuming too much potassium can lead to hyperkalemia—higher than normal blood levels of the mineral [15]. Fortunately, the risk of the condition is practically non-existent in healthy people following a balanced diet. Even if you consume more of the mineral, your body can readily excrete excess amounts through urine.

Supplementation can increase the risk of potassium toxicity, but the condition is rare even in such a scenario. The person would have to take way more than the recommended amount for many days in a row to reach dangerous blood levels.

People in certain situations or with specific conditions could be more likely to develop hyperkalemia. Here are some risk factors [16]:

- Going through chemotherapy
- Having diabetes
- Suffering from kidney disease
- Overtraining for prolonged periods

- Taking potassium-conserving diuretics
- Using cocaine

Arrhythmia (abnormal heart rhythm) is the most common symptom of too much potassium. In rare cases, toxicity can result in death [16].

FINAL THOUGHTS

Potassium is arguably among the most important nutrients you need for optimal health, well-being, energy levels, and athleticism.

One of the mineral's most notable functions relates to fluid balance. Potassium is necessary for regulating intracellular and extracellular fluid volume, along with the total fluid volume in your body.

Getting enough potassium can improve nerve signalling, regulate blood pressure, improve muscle contractions, and even reduce the risk of osteoporosis later in life.

While many people provide at least some amount of the mineral, folks struggle to get enough potassium and are at risk of a mild deficiency.

REFERENCES

1. www.ncbi.nlm.nih.gov/books/NBK539791/
2. www.ncbi.nlm.nih.gov/books/NBK442010/
3. www.ncbi.nlm.nih.gov/books/NBK279390/
4. www.ncbi.nlm.nih.gov/pmc/articles/PMC2929932/
5. www.pubmed.ncbi.nlm.nih.gov/18653669/
6. www.ncbi.nlm.nih.gov/pmc/articles/PMC8989702/
7. www.cdc.gov/bloodpressure/facts.htm
8. www.pubmed.ncbi.nlm.nih.gov/23558164/
9. www.ncbi.nlm.nih.gov/books/NBK441901/
10. www.pubmed.ncbi.nlm.nih.gov/15817873/
11. www.pubmed.ncbi.nlm.nih.gov/10617959/
12. www.ncbi.nlm.nih.gov/pmc/articles/PMC5685519/
13. www.ncbi.nlm.nih.gov/pmc/articles/PMC4525130/
14. www.ods.od.nih.gov/factsheets/Potassium-Consumer
15. www.ncbi.nlm.nih.gov/books/NBK470284/
16. www.ncbi.nlm.nih.gov/pmc/articles/PMC6892421/

ZINC

Numerous nutrients play an important role in our health. Among these, we have protein, dietary fats, and various vitamins and minerals.

Zinc is one essential nutrient involved in many biological processes. The nutrient is found in every cell and plays a crucial role in the optimal functioning of the human body.

Today's guide will cover what zinc is, how it promotes good health, how to get enough of it daily, and much more.

WHAT IS ZINC?

Zinc is one of the 14 essential minerals your body needs to sustain itself. The mineral is the second most abundant in your body (after iron) and is found in every cell.

Similar to magnesium, zinc plays a role in numerous bodily processes. It is involved in over 300 biological processes related to protein synthesis, DNA repair, gene expression, growth, development, immunity, nerve function, and more [1].

Like all other minerals and most vitamins (excluding A, D, E, and K), zinc is water-soluble. The nutrient dissolves in water, and your body readily excretes excess amounts. Because of that, you must get enough zinc through food and supplements every day.

The great news is that zinc occurs naturally in a wide range of foods (more on that below), so the risk of a deficiency is relatively low for healthy individuals.

Interestingly, a potential symptom of low zinc levels could be a reduction in your senses of taste and smell because the mineral is crucial for producing an enzyme necessary for both [2].

Zinc is often added to formulas designed to boost immunity, medications like nasal sprays, and drugs for the common cold.

WHAT FUNCTIONS DOES ZINC HAVE IN THE BODY?

1. Necessary for Immune System Health

Similar to vitamin C, zinc is well-known for its immunity-boosting properties. The mineral is crucial for the optimal functioning of cells and for the communication between parts of the immune system. A zinc deficiency can increase the susceptibility to various pathogens [3].

First, zinc appears crucial for skin barrier integrity [3]. Adequate zinc levels are necessary to prevent external invaders from entering your body.

Second, zinc is necessary for the gene expression within lymphocytes (a type of white blood cell) and supports the function of neutrophils and natural killer cells that destroy external invaders and keep you healthy [3].

The mineral also possesses antioxidant functions and can protect healthy cells from oxidative stress [4].

One review noted that zinc supplementation could shorten the common cold duration by 2.25 days in healthy adults [5]. Further, research shows that adequate zinc levels are necessary for optimal immune system function in aging adults [6].

2. May Promote Wound Healing

Collagen is the most abundant protein in the human body, accounting for 25 to 35 percent of the total protein in your body [7]. The protein is found in almost all tissues, including skeletal muscle, connective tissues, and the skin.

Zinc plays a vital role in collagen synthesis and is often used as part of treatment for burns and other skin injuries [8]. According to research, your skin holds up to five percent of all zinc in your body [9].

A zinc deficiency can slow wound healing, and supplementation can speed up the process [8]. For example, in one study of 60 subjects with diabetic foot ulcers, zinc supplementation significantly reduced ulcer size compared to placebo [10].

3. Could Be Helpful Against Acne

Acne might not seem like that big of an issue, but the skin condition affects millions of people and often contributes to social anxiety, depression, and low self-esteem [11].

According to some statistics, acne affects between 40 and 50 million people in the US, including children and adults over 25 [12].

As mentioned in the previous point, the skin holds up to five percent of the zinc found in the body. Interestingly, the mineral can also help treat acne and lower the risk of recurrence.

Research shows that zinc supplements can improve skin texture and reduce the risk of acne [13]. For example, one paper suggests that zinc sulfate can be a viable alternative to traditional acne treatment in people with moderate to severe acne [14].

Zinc can also be used as a first step to battling acne and other skin problems because the supplement is inexpensive, effective, and far less likely to bring any side effects.

4. Reduces Inflammation (And Can Lower the Risk of Some Conditions)

Inflammation is your body's response to infections, harmful bacteria, viruses, and more. It's an immune system response that keeps you healthy.

Unfortunately, inflammation isn't always helpful and can sometimes do more harm than good.

Chronic inflammation is a long-lasting immune system response. It can last for weeks, months, or even years, long after the initial threat is no longer around. The problem is that elevated inflammatory markers can put a person at a higher risk of various conditions, including cancer [15].

The good news is that zinc can reduce levels of certain inflammatory proteins [16]. In one paper, researchers noted that zinc supplementation could decrease lipid peroxidation, inflammatory cytokines, and C-reactive protein [17].

5. Could Be Good for Cardiovascular Health

Cardiovascular health depends on numerous factors, including activity level, diet, sleep, and stress. Leading a healthier lifestyle is the most crucial step to protecting your heart and reducing the risk of numerous health issues.

Interestingly, zinc could help improve several risk factors for cardiovascular disease. First, zinc can have a favorable impact on blood triglyceride and cholesterol levels. In one review from 2015, researchers looked at 24 studies on the matter and found that zinc supplementation can reduce LDL (bad) cholesterol and triglyceride levels [18].

Second, zinc can have favorable effects on blood pressure. A review of nine studies found that zinc supplementation can significantly reduce systolic blood pressure [19]. Systolic blood pressure measures the pressure in your arteries when your heart beats.

High blood pressure is a considerable risk factor for cardiovascular disease; finding ways to manage it is necessary to maintain a healthy heart.

Additionally, as discussed earlier, zinc can have antioxidant and anti-inflammatory effects on the body. Controlling oxidative stress and inflammation is vital for cardiovascular health [20].

HOW MUCH ZINC DO YOU NEED, AND WHAT ARE SOME GOOD SOURCES?

Here is the recommended daily zinc intake based on age [21]:

- First six months - 2 mg
- 7 months to three years - 3 mg
- 4 to 8 years - 5 mg
- 9 to 13 years - 8 mg
- 14 to 18 years - 11 mg (boys) and 9 mg (girls)
- 19+ years - 11 mg (men) and 8 mg (women)

Pregnant and lactating women should consume 11 to 13 mg of zinc daily. Here is a list of some great dietary zinc sources:

- Oysters - just two medium-sized oysters cover all of your daily needs
- Ground beef - 43 percent of daily needs per 3.5 ounces
- Dark chocolate - up to 30 percent of daily needs per 3.5 ounces
- Cashews - 15 percent of daily needs per ounce
- Lentils - 11 percent of daily needs per 3.5 ounces
- Potato - 10 percent of daily needs per large potato
- Hemp seeds - 9 percent of daily needs per tablespoon
- Whole milk - 9 percent of daily needs per cup
- Eggs - 5 percent of daily needs per large egg

It's important to note that legumes (lentils, beans, etc.) contain phytates, which can inhibit the absorption of zinc and other minerals [22]. So, it's best to serve these foods in moderation and consume more animal products to get enough zinc daily.

IS THERE A RISK OF ZINC DEFICIENCY, AND WHAT ARE SOME SYMPTOMS?

A zinc deficiency is unlikely to occur in healthy people following a moderately-balanced diet. The nutrient is found in many whole foods, and it's not that challenging to cover your daily needs.

Still, it's essential to be mindful of your food choices because your body readily excretes excess amounts, so you must get the nutrient daily.

Following a vegan diet can increase your risk of a zinc deficiency because [23]:

a. It can be more challenging to get enough zinc
b. The phytates found in plant foods can impact zinc absorption

Excessive dieting and alcohol abuse can also increase the risk of zinc deficiency.

People with zinc deficiency often experience [2]:

- Hair loss and thinning
- Impaired testosterone production and low libido
- Loss of appetite
- Eye and vision problems
- Irritability

HOW HIGH IS THE RISK OF ZINC TOXICITY, AND SHOULD YOU WORRY?

Zinc toxicity is unlikely in healthy people following a balanced diet. People at risk of toxicity are those supplementing with large doses or using denture adhesive creams that contain zinc.

Some common symptoms of too much zinc include [24]:

- Appetite loss
- Nausea and vomiting
- Dizziness
- GI issues

Taking too much zinc can also interfere with copper absorption, leading to impaired immune system function and low HDL (good) cholesterol [25].

CONCLUSION

Zinc is a mineral involved in numerous bodily processes, including immunity, metabolism, DNA synthesis, and development.

Some data finds that zinc can reduce the risk of health issues related to oxidative stress and inflammation.

The good news is that a zinc deficiency is unlikely for healthy people following a balanced diet.

REFERENCES

1. www.ncbi.nlm.nih.gov/pmc/articles/PMC2820120/

2. www.ncbi.nlm.nih.gov/books/NBK493231/

3. www.pubmed.ncbi.nlm.nih.gov/9701160/

4. www.pubmed.ncbi.nlm.nih.gov/28083748/

5. www.ncbi.nlm.nih.gov/pmc/articles/PMC7356429/

6. www.ncbi.nlm.nih.gov/pmc/articles/PMC2702361/

7. www.ncbi.nlm.nih.gov/pmc/articles/PMC2846778/

8. www.ncbi.nlm.nih.gov/pmc/articles/PMC3188105/

9. www.ncbi.nlm.nih.gov/pmc/articles/PMC5793244/

10. www.pubmed.ncbi.nlm.nih.gov/28395131/

11. www.ncbi.nlm.nih.gov/pmc/articles/PMC3051295/

12. www.jamanetwork.com/journals/jamadermatology/fullarticle/479093

13. www.pubmed.ncbi.nlm.nih.gov/29193602/

14. www.pubmed.ncbi.nlm.nih.gov/34188751/

15. www.ncbi.nlm.nih.gov/pmc/articles/PMC7147972/

16. www.ncbi.nlm.nih.gov/pmc/articles/PMC4469681/

17. www.ncbi.nlm.nih.gov/pmc/articles/PMC2869512/

18. www.ncbi.nlm.nih.gov/pmc/articles/PMC4523910/

19. www.pubmed.ncbi.nlm.nih.gov/32090294/

20. www.ncbi.nlm.nih.gov/pmc/articles/PMC3157078/

21. www.ods.od.nih.gov/factsheets/Zinc-HealthProfessional/

22. www.pubmed.ncbi.nlm.nih.gov/32987890/

23. www.ncbi.nlm.nih.gov/pmc/articles/PMC7073751/

24. www.ncbi.nlm.nih.gov/books/NBK554548/

25. www.pubmed.ncbi.nlm.nih.gov/20617034/

SODIUM

Sodium is a nutrient almost everyone consumes daily. But how much do you know about it and its effects on your body?

Today's guide will cover all things sodium by going over its impact on your health, some potential dangers, and tips for optimal consumption.

Let's dive in.

WHAT IS SODIUM?

Sodium, better known as salt, is an essential mineral your body needs to carry out certain vital processes [1]. The mineral occurs naturally in many foods and drinks and is often used as a flavoring agent.

Like all other essential minerals and most vitamins, sodium is water-soluble. It dissolves in liquids, and your body can remove some of it through urination and sweat.

Unfortunately, that doesn't mean you should ignore your sodium intake. Unlike other minerals, sodium overconsumption isn't as difficult, especially if you enjoy canned goods, processed foods, etc. Even non-salty foods like cereal can contain sodium and increase your daily intake.

Let's now explore what functions sodium has in the body, what risks overconsumption brings, and how much you should get each day.

WHAT ARE SODIUM'S FUNCTIONS IN THE BODY?

1. It Functions as An Electrolyte

Sodium is one of six electrolytes (along with potassium, phosphate, calcium, chloride, and magnesium) your body needs to function optimally [1, 2].

Electrolytes function by releasing a positive or negative charge when dissolved in water. These electrical impulses are necessary for regulating various chemical reactions, promoting nerve signalling, maintaining fluid balance, and more [2].

Sodium is one of the most important electrolytes because it serves two functions. First, it regulates fluid balance (we'll look at this next). Second, it allows cells to absorb the nutrients they need to function optimally.

Additionally, sodium is necessary for optimal brain and muscle function [3]. While it alone doesn't ensure or prevent optimal bodily functioning, a deficiency (hyponatremia) can lead to muscle weakness, confusion, impaired reflexes, nausea, etc. [4].

2. It Is Necessary for Fluid Balance

One of sodium's most notable functions relates to fluid balance, which refers to two things:
- The amount of fluid your body maintains
- The balance between intracellular and extracellular fluids

Research shows that the adult human body is 60 percent water [5]. Almost half is intracellular fluid (found within your body's cells), and the remaining is extracellular fluid (located outside the body's cells).

Sodium is one of the two electrolytes (along with potassium) necessary for maintaining the balance between intracellular and extracellular fluid. Specifically, sodium is responsible for regulating the amount of extracellular fluid, and potassium maintains healthy fluid levels within cells. The objective is to have similar fluid levels inside and outside cells.

Too little or too much sodium can impact the balance.

3. It Plays an Important Role In Cardiovascular Health

Cardiovascular disease is the leading cause of death worldwide. According to statistics, one person in the United States dies of cardiovascular-related issues every 34 seconds, amounting to 697,000 deaths annually [6].

While numerous studies link a high sodium intake to cardiovascular disease, not getting enough can be equally dangerous. In one review with over 133,000 participants, researchers looked at the relationship between sodium intake and cardiovascular disease (CVD) risk [7].

According to their findings, people who consumed less than 3,000 mg (3 grams) of sodium daily were at a higher risk of CVD and early death. In contrast, those consuming 4,000 to 5,000 mg daily were more likely to stay healthy and live longer.

Another study had similar findings [8]. In it, researchers examined more than 101,000 participants and followed up with them nearly four years later. According to their results, people consuming 3,000 to 6,000 mg of sodium daily were at a much lower risk of death and cardiovascular events.

4. It Regulates Blood Pressure

A common argument against sodium is that it leads to hypertension, which is linked to cardiovascular disease, a higher risk of heart attack, and early death [9, 10]. These effects appear particularly pronounced in people already struggling with elevated blood pressure.

While that can be the case in some people, it isn't always true. For instance, some data suggests that not getting enough sodium can have the opposite effect: low blood pressure (hypotension) [4].

Low blood pressure is less harmful than hypertension, but there are still risks. Most notably, hypotension can lead to dizziness, nausea, blurred vision, and, in severe cases, fainting [4].

People struggling with low blood pressure should be particularly mindful of their sodium intake and avoid unnecessary restrictions.

HOW MUCH SODIUM SHOULD YOU GET EACH DAY?

One of the most common recommendations is to limit sodium intake. But, as we saw in the previous point, that could come with some issues.

The question is, how much sodium should you get for optimal health? Unlike the recommendations we see for other minerals, the optimal sodium intake seems less clear and dependent on more factors.

For example, some sources recommend limiting sodium to 2,300 mg daily to avoid hypertension and the associated dangers. But, as we saw in some papers above, a higher intake can reduce the risk of cardiovascular disease and early death [7, 8].

A good approach is to consume sodium based on your circumstances. For example, if you're someone who has historically suffered from hypertension or the condition runs in your family, perhaps limiting your intake would be healthier in the long run.

In contrast, people with normal blood pressure and no family history of cardiovascular disease could be a bit more liberal with their intake. Similarly, if your blood pressure runs on the low end, it may be better to consume at least 3,000 mg of sodium daily.

In any case, these are just recommendations and should not be taken as medical advice. It's best to consult your healthcare provider and follow their recommendations, especially if you're dealing with a condition.

IS THERE A RISK OF CONSUMING TOO MUCH SODIUM (AND WHAT ARE THE RISKS)?

Your body needs sodium to function optimally, but there is a risk of overconsumption, especially for people eating too many processed and canned foods.

Here are two potential problems related to excess sodium intake:

1. Hypertension and Cardiovascular Disease

One of the biggest dangers of sodium overconsumption is hypertension, which is linked to cardiovascular disease and a higher risk of heart attack and stroke. High blood pressure is often called the silent killer because it can come with minor symptoms but damage blood vessels and other tissues in the body.

Some research also links hypertension to cognitive impairment and a higher risk of neurodegenerative diseases [11].

For example, in one literature review, researchers looked at sodium intake and health outcomes in people with and without hypertension [12]. With over 133,000 participants across the examined studies, the authors noted a strong correlation between higher sodium intake, cardiovascular disease risk, and early death.

Another review examined over 229,000 participants across 11 studies [13]. The average follow-up period was 13.37 years. Data again suggested that higher sodium intake is linked to an increased risk of early death due to cardiovascular problems.

A more recent review of the literature looked at nearly 618,000 people, suggesting that every gram of sodium increases the risk of cardiovascular disease by six percent [14].

2. Potentially Higher Stomach Cancer Risk

Stomach cancer is a common form of the disease and one of the leading causes of cancer-related deaths today. It accounts for just over 11,000 annual deaths in the US [15].

As with other conditions, numerous factors can increase the risk of stomach cancer. Some data suggests that excess sodium intake is one risk factor.

For instance, one paper shows that people with a strong preference for saltier foods are more likely to develop stomach cancer than those who consume salt sparingly [16]. Data comes from a lifestyle questionnaire completed by nearly 41,000 Japanese adults aged 40 to 79.

One hypothesis is that excess sodium intake creates a positive environment for Helicobacter pylori (H. pylori). The bacteria increases the risk of inflammation, stomach ulcers, and cancer [17].

We need more research on the topic, and none of the studies claim that sodium leads to stomach cancer. These are merely correlations.

HOW TO OPTIMIZE YOUR SODIUM INTAKE
1. Avoid Salty Foods

Some foods are jam-packed with sodium, and just a few servings can provide several grams of sodium.

Be careful with:
- Canned goods
- Microwave popcorn
- Crackers, chips, etc.
- Frozen meals
- Pickles
- Soy sauce

2. Try Before Adding Salt

Some people have the bad habit of adding salt to meals before trying the food. Get rid of the practice by making it a point to sample a meal before adding salt.

Ask yourself, "Does the meal genuinely need extra salt, or can I enjoy it as it is?"

3. Try Salt Alternatives

Who says the only way to cook and make meals tastier is by adding salt? There are plenty of great alternatives to experiment with:
- Black and red pepper
- Garlic
- Apple cider vinegar
- Onion powder
- Rosemary
- Sage

FINAL WORDS

Sodium is an essential mineral your body needs for fluid balance, cardiovascular health, and more.

Unfortunately, excess sodium consumption can increase the risk of health issues, including cardiovascular disease.

It's important to be mindful of your sodium intake, especially if you have hypertension or the condition runs in your family.

REFERENCES

1. www.ncbi.nlm.nih.gov/pmc/articles/PMC3951800/
2. www.ncbi.nlm.nih.gov/books/NBK541123/
3. www.ncbi.nlm.nih.gov/pmc/articles/PMC5334786/
4. www.ncbi.nlm.nih.gov/books/NBK470386/
5. www.ncbi.nlm.nih.gov/pmc/articles/PMC2929932/
6. www.cdc.gov/heartdisease/facts.htm
7. www.pubmed.ncbi.nlm.nih.gov/27216139/
8. www.pubmed.ncbi.nlm.nih.gov/25119607/
9. www.ncbi.nlm.nih.gov/pmc/articles/PMC6770596/
10. www.pubmed.ncbi.nlm.nih.gov/31865786/
11. www.ncbi.nlm.nih.gov/pmc/articles/PMC8031190/
12. www.pubmed.ncbi.nlm.nih.gov/27216139/
13. www.pubmed.ncbi.nlm.nih.gov/24848764/
14. www.pubmed.ncbi.nlm.nih.gov/32992705/
15. www.cancer.org/cancer/stomach-cancer/about/key-statistics.html
16. www.ncbi.nlm.nih.gov/pmc/articles/PMC4728120/
17. www.pubmed.ncbi.nlm.nih.gov/32861308/

OMEGA 3,6 AND 9

O mega 3, 6, and 9 fatty acids are dietary components with various essential functions in the body. These nutrients also interact with one another and sometimes even compete for a spot inside cells.

Today's guide will outline the three forms of dietary fat, their unique functions, and how they impact your health. We will also share some excellent food sources.

Let's dive in.

A BRIEF LOOK AT DIETARY FAT STRUCTURE

Before diving into the various fatty acids you should consume, we have to take a brief look at their chemical structures. That information will make everything else much easier to understand.

There are three primary types of fatty acids [1]:

- Monounsaturated fats
- Polyunsaturated fats
- Saturated fats

Each type of fat has a unique chemical formula that determines how it gets metabolized and what impact it has on your body [1]. Monounsaturated fats are molecules with one unsaturated carbon bond, also known as a double bond.

Polyunsaturated fats are molecules with more than one unsaturated carbon bond in their structure. In contrast, saturated fats have no double bonds.

WHAT ARE OMEGA 3 FATTY ACIDS (AND WHAT FUNCTIONS DO THEY HAVE)?

Omega-3 fatty acids are a form of polyunsaturated fats your body cannot produce, hence their status as 'essential.' In other words, you must get enough of them from your diet [2].

The three omega-3 fatty acids are docosahexaenoic acid (DHA), eicosapentaenoic acid (EPA), and alpha-linolenic acid (ALA). DHA and EPA are primarily found in animal foods and algae, whereas ALA occurs naturally in plant foods.

Good food sources of these three fatty acids include fatty fish (salmon, mackerel, trout, etc.), fish oil, flaxseeds, flaxseed oil, chia seeds, and some nuts.

An omega-3 fatty acid supplement can benefit people who don't eat many of these foods, especially fish.

Let's now take a look at the three fatty acids:

EPA

Eicosapentaenoic acid is a fatty acid mostly found in fish and fish oil. Part of it can get converted to DHA when your body needs it.

Taking EPA is vital for maintaining cardiovascular health and reducing the risk of heart attack and stroke [3].

Researchers have also explored the effectiveness of EPA for people with conditions like schizophrenia, Alzheimer's, attention deficit hyperactivity disorder (ADHD), depression, and more [4, 5].

The fatty acid also appears beneficial for eye health and vision in older adults [6]. Regular consumption can slow down age-related macular degradation (AMD), allowing people to maintain their vision longer.

Some research suggests that EPA can be beneficial for people with cancer. The fatty acid can reduce the side effects of chemotherapy [7].

Like other nutrients, EPA also appears necessary during pregnancy [8]. The fatty acid can promote a healthy pregnancy by normalizing blood pressure and reducing the risk of fetal growth restriction (FGR).

DHA

Docosahexaenoic acid (DHA) is similar to EPA. The fatty acid is also found in fatty fish and fish oil and has similar health functions.

One of the fatty acid's crucial functions relates to pregnancy. DHA begins to accumulate in the brain during pregnancy, and levels continue to rise during the first two years of life [9]. Because of that, women are advised to take a fish oil supplement containing at least 200 mg of DHA during their pregnancy.

Brain levels of the fatty acid remain mostly the same after the first two years and maintaining them depends on healthy food choices or regular supplementation.

Research suggests that low DHA consumption can lead to memory loss, mood swings, difficulty concentrating, and a higher risk of neurodegenerative disorders like Alzheimer's [10].

ALA

Alpha-lipoic acid (ALA) is the third omega-3 fatty acid. Unlike EPA and DHA, ALA is mainly found in plants, and you don't necessarily have to eat fatty fish or algae to maintain optimal levels.

One notable function of ALA is its antioxidant ability [11]. The fatty acid is found in all human cells, and research suggests that it can protect healthy cells from reactive oxygen species (ROS).

ALA is unique because your body can produce some amounts when needed. It gets made in the mitochondria (the powerhouse of the cells) and helps the body produce energy.

A unique benefit of ALA is that it is water- and fat-soluble, which allows it to impact every cell in the body. In contrast, most antioxidants are water or fat-soluble.

Research also links ALA to reduced risk of diabetes, improved memory and cognition, weight loss, skin health, and anti-inflammatory effects [11, 12].

Excellent Food Sources of Omega-3 Fatty Acids

- Caviar - 6,000+ mg of combined EPA and DHA per 3.5 ounces
- Chia seeds - 5,000+ mg of ALA per ounce
- Mackerel - 4,600 mg of combined EPA and DHA per 3.5 ounces
- Walnuts - 2,570 mg of ALA per ounce
- Flaxseeds - 2,300+ mg of ALA per tablespoon
- Salmon - 2,150 mg of combined EPA and DHA per 3.5 ounces
- Herring - 2,150 mg of combined EPA and DHA per 3.5 ounces
- Sardines - 1,460 mg of combined EPA and DHA per 3.5 ounces
- Soybeans - 1,400+ mg of ALA per 3.5 ounces
- Oysters - 390 mg of combined EPA and DHA per 3.5 ounces

WHAT ARE OMEGA 6 FATTY ACIDS (AND WHY ARE THEY IMPORTANT)?

Similar to omega-3 fatty acids, omega-6 are polyunsaturated, though there are some differences in their chemical structures. Omega-6 fatty acids are also essential because your body cannot produce them, and you must get them through food.

A common omega-6 fatty acid is linoleic acid (LA). Your body can convert LA to longer-chain fatty acids like arachidonic acid (AA).

Unlike omega-3 fatty acids, omega-6 are much easier to obtain from food because they are found in vegetable oils, nuts, seeds, and more. Meat from animals raised in factories is also a good source of omega-6 fatty acids because the diet of such animals mostly consists of corn and soy.

Omega 3 and 6 Fatty Acids in Balance

An adequate omega-6 fatty acid intake is necessary for good health, but there must be a balance with your omega-3 intake. According to research, the ideal ratio between omega-3 and omega-6 fatty acids is between 1:1 and 1:4 [13]. Unfortunately, the Western diet has shifted that ratio to 1:15 or more.

Increasing your omega-3 intake is necessary because the two classes of fatty acids fight for a place in cell membranes. Some researchers suggest that maintaining a healthy ratio is far more critical than the absolute amount of fat you consume [13].

The cells in your body have a lipid bilayer—a structure with two layers of fat that envelops your cells. These 'barriers' serve the crucial function of determining what goes in and out of your cells.

Consuming more omega-3 fatty acids leads to more fluid cell barriers that allow neurochemicals and other compounds to enter your cells. In contrast, consuming mostly omega-6 fatty acids and not enough omega-3s leads to more rigid membranes, preventing helpful compounds from entering.

Foods Rich In Omega-6 Fats

- Walnuts - 10,000+ mg of LA per ounce
- Sunflower seeds - 10,000+ mg of LA per ounce
- Tofu - 6,000+ mg of LA per 3.5 ounces
- Almonds - 3,400+ mg of LA per ounce
- Hemp seeds - 2,700+ mg of LA per tablespoon
- Cashews - 2,200+ mg of LA per ounce
- Peanut butter - 1,900 mg of LA per tablespoon

- Safflower oil - 1,700+ mg of LA per tablespoon
- Avocado oil - 1,700+ mg of LA per tablespoon
- Eggs - 600 mg of LA per large egg

The great thing is that your body can convert linoleic acid (LA) to longer-chain fats, depending on what your body needs.

WHAT ARE OMEGA 9 FATTY ACIDS (AND WHY YOUR BODY NEEDS THEM)

Unlike omega-3 and omega-6 fatty acids, omega-9 are monounsaturated: having one double bond. Oleic acid is the most popular omega-9 fat and the most common monounsaturated fatty acid in most people's diets.

Another difference is that omega-9 fats aren't essential because your body can synthesize them when needed. Still, getting some omega-9 fats from your diet can offer several health benefits.

For example, in one large observational study, researchers looked at the link between monounsaturated fatty acid (MUFA) intake and cardiovascular disease risk among more than 63,000 women and almost 30,000 men [14].

Researchers noted that consuming more MUFAs from plant sources was correlated with a lower risk of coronary heart disease.

Further, data suggests that monounsaturated fats can lower LDL (bad) cholesterol and potentially increase HDL (good) cholesterol [15].

Foods That Provide Omega-9 Fats

- Macadamia nuts - 12,600 mg of oleic acid per ounce
- Sunflower oils - 11,000+ mg of oleic acid per tablespoon
- Almonds - 11,000+ mg of oleic acid per ounce
- Argan oil - 3,400+ mg of oleic acid per tablespoon
- Peanut butter - 5,700+ mg of oleic acid per ounce
- Chia seeds - 800+ mg of oleic acid per ounce

FINAL WORDS

As you can see, all three types of Omega fatty acids play an important role in our health and longevity.

Most people can get enough Omega 6 and 9 fatty acids through food, but that's not always the case for omega-3 (especially EPA and DHA).

Eating various fat-rich foods, including fatty fish, is the best way to get enough of the numerous fats your body needs. A fish oil supplement can also be useful for getting a concentrated dose of EPA and DHA.

REFERENCES

1. www.ncbi.nlm.nih.gov/pmc/articles/PMC4190204/
2. www.ncbi.nlm.nih.gov/pmc/articles/PMC3262608/
3. www.pubmed.ncbi.nlm.nih.gov/24047614/
4. www.pubmed.ncbi.nlm.nih.gov/20439549/
5. www.pubmed.ncbi.nlm.nih.gov/14623502/
6. www.ncbi.nlm.nih.gov/books/NBK11888/
7. www.ncbi.nlm.nih.gov/pmc/articles/PMC6566772/
8. www.ncbi.nlm.nih.gov/pmc/articles/PMC3046737/
9. www.ncbi.nlm.nih.gov/pmc/articles/PMC2647754/
10. www.ncbi.nlm.nih.gov/pmc/articles/PMC4772061/
11. www.ncbi.nlm.nih.gov/pmc/articles/PMC6594273/
12. www.ncbi.nlm.nih.gov/pmc/articles/PMC5732919/
13. www.pubmed.ncbi.nlm.nih.gov/12442909/
14. www.ncbi.nlm.nih.gov/pmc/articles/PMC5875103/
15. www.ncbi.nlm.nih.gov/pmc/articles/PMC3546618/

Printed in Great Britain
by Amazon

35094726R00076